THE ULTIMATE KETTLEBELL WORKBOOK

DISCARD
Centerville Library
Washington-Centerville
Centerville, Ohio

W9-BNX-535

THE ULTIMATE KETTLEBELL WORKBOOK

THE REVOLUTIONARY PROGRAM TO TONE, SCULPT AND STRENGTHEN YOUR WHOLE BODY

DAVE RANDOLPH

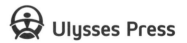 Ulysses Press

Text Copyright © 2011 Dave Randolph. Design and Concept © 2011 Ulysses Press and its licensors. Photographs copyright © 2011 Rapt Productions except as noted below. All rights reserved. No part of this publication may be reproduced, stored in a retrieval system, or transmitted in any form or by any means without the prior written permission of the publisher, nor be otherwise circulated in any form of binding or cover other than that in which it is published and without a similar condition being imposed on the subsequent purchaser.

Published in the United States by
Ulysses Press
P.O. Box 3440
Berkeley, CA 94703
www.ulyssespress.com

ISBN: 978-1-56975-874-8
Library of Congress Control Number 2010937126

Printed in Canada by Webcom

10 9 8 7 6 5 4 3 2 1

Acquisitions: Keith Riegert
Managing editor: Claire Chun
Editor: Lily Chou
Proofreader: Lauren Harrison
Production: Judith Metzener
Index: Sayre Van Young
Cover design: what!design @ whatweb.com
Cover and interior photographs: © Rapt Productions except page 12 © lienedizenberga/Fotolia.com
Models: Michael Espero, Fernando Felix, Meredith Miller, Miriam Nakamoto, Dave Randolph

Distributed by Publishers Group West

Please Note
This book has been written and published strictly for informational purposes, and in no way should be used as a substitute for actual instruction with qualified professionals. The author and publisher are providing you with information in this work so that you can have the knowledge and can choose, at your own risk, to act on that knowledge. The author and publisher also urge all readers to be aware of their health status and to consult health care professionals before beginning any health program.

Table of Contents

PART 1: GETTING STARTED

Introduction 8

History of Kettlebells 9

Benefits of Kettlebell Training 11

Before You Begin 12

PART 2: THE PROGRAMS

How to Use This Book 16

Designing Your Own Program 17

Workout 1: Scaled Exercises for Beginner/
  Intermediate/Advanced 24

Workout 2: Beginner General
  Conditioning 26

Workout 3: Beginner Strength 28

Workout 4: Intermediate Strength 29

Workout 5: Intermediate General
  Conditioning 30

Workout 6: Advanced Strength 31

Workout 7: Advanced Conditioning 31

Workout 8: Advanced Power Plus
  Conditioning 32

Workout 9: Strength—As Heavy As
  Possible 33

Workout 10: Conditioning—All Levels 34

PART 3: THE EXERCISES

Swing Progression 38

Sumo Deadlift 40

Two-Hand Swing 42

One-Hand Swing 43

Hand-to-Hand (H2H) Swing 45

Hand-to-Hand (H2H) Swing with Release 46

High Pull 47

Double Swing 48

Cleans Progression 49

One-Arm Vertical High Pull (1AVHP) 51

Dead Clean 52

Hang Clean 54

Pendulum Clean 55

Double Dead Clean 56

Double Hang Clean 57

Double Pendulum Clean 58

Overhead Press 59

Overhead Press 60

Push Press 62

Deadlift Progression 64

Suitcase Deadlift 65

One-Leg Suitcase Deadlift 66

Stiff-Legged One-Leg Deadlift 68

Squat Progression 70

Sumo Squat 71

Goblet Squat 72

Front Squat 74

Floor Press 75

Rows 77

Slingshots 78

Figure 8s 79

Figure 8 79

Figure 8 with a Tap 80

Renegade Row   82

Snatches   83

    Dead Snatch   86

    Hang Snatch   88

    Pendulum Snatch   89

Alternating Cleans   91

    Two-Step Alternating Clean   92

    One-Step Alternating Clean   93

Turkish Getups   94

    Half Getup   96

    Turkish Getup   98

    Getup Sit-Up   101

    Armbar   102

Windmills   103

    Low Windmill   104

    Overhead Windmill   105

    Double Windmill   106

Jerks   107

    One-Arm Jerk   108

PART 4: APPENDIX

Warm-Ups   112

Cool-Downs   129

References   137

Index   138

Acknowledgments   143

About the Author   144

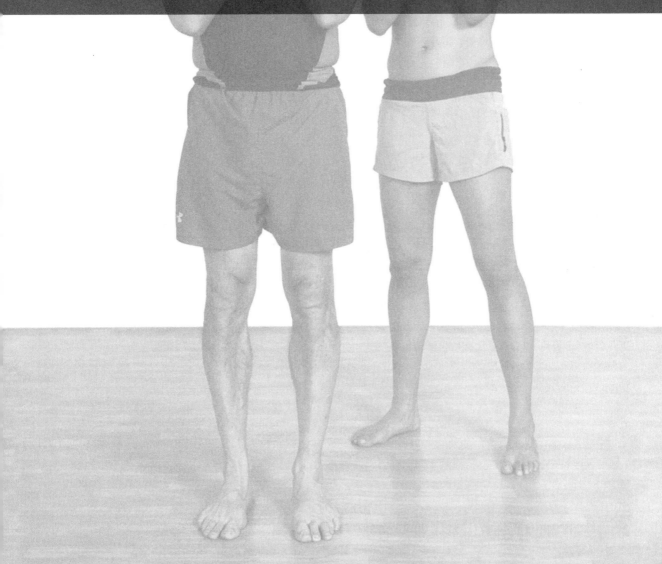

PART 1

GETTING STARTED

Introduction

Are you stuck in an exercise rut, spending hours at the gym, bored to tears on the treadmill? Tired of waiting in line for a machine or trying to use the squat rack while someone is playing around in it doing 30-pound barbell curls? Have you been doing the same routine for months or years on end and have stopped seeing any progress? Or maybe you're just looking to introduce a new tool into your fitness arsenal?

If you've answered "yes" to any of these questions, then welcome to *The Ultimate Kettlebell Workbook*. You're about to enter the fun, fast-paced world of kettlebell training for fat loss, general fitness, flexibility and mobility, as well as sports performance and enhancement.

Since I started training with kettlebells in 2002, I've seen big differences in my own body's composition as well as those of my clients: less fat and more muscle. In addition, improved hand and foot speed, reaction time, conditioning, strength and power have made everyday tasks like yard work and climbing stairs much easier. When shoveling snow after a blizzard, one 50-year-old client realized that his conditioning was better than it was when he was 30. Clients who participate in equestrian events have found that they ride much better than before they started kettlebell training. Avid tennis players report improved performance in foot, hand and reaction speed as well as the ability to hit the ball harder and more accurately.

This book will teach you how to use kettlebells safely and effectively to transform your current fitness regimen into a dynamic, high-intensity workout that will help you get the body you want with less time in the gym (which means more time for other things). You'll learn the proper way to do the primary lifts and variations, as well as how to add them into your current workout or use them to replace your current workout completely.

No matter what your fitness goals are, kettlebell training will make you stronger, improve your endurance and enhance your core strength.

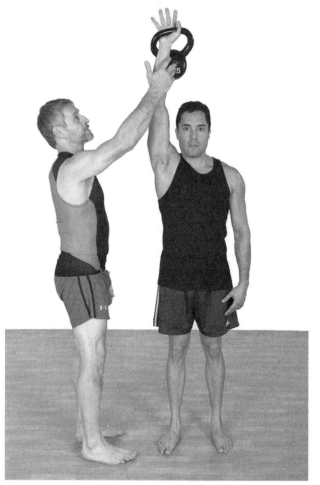

Author Dave Randolph makes some adjustments.

History of Kettlebells

Kettlebells, which are Russian in origin (called *girya*), are believed to have been around since the early 1700s. They were originally used as a measure of weight called a *pood* (about 16 kilograms, or 35 pounds). A farmer would bring in his crop, which would then be put on a scale and weighed against the *girya*. Eventually, perhaps sometime in the mid-1800s, someone started tossing *girya* around and decided it would make a great exercise tool.

Many photographs from the late 1800s and early 1900s feature old-time strong men wielding kettlebells of various sizes and shapes. In fact, kettlebells were used quite a bit back in the days before bodybuilding came into vogue. In those days, men lifted weights to get stronger and gain a lean, athletic physique, like that of a Greek or Roman statue. They didn't want big bulky muscles and a V-taper—they knew that shape was not functionally strong. In addition, big muscles require more food and energy to maintain and also make it harder to move. By working on pure strength and power, the weight lifters of that time became strong and lean, with a thick, solid core. They were proportional and had tremendous strength that they used in everyday life.

When bodybuilding became popular in the 1940s, people tended toward big chests and biceps and began neglecting the back of their body. They wanted to look strong but neglected the muscles that actually make you strong, training the muscles that can be seen in a mirror instead of those in the rear.

Things got even worse in the late 1960s with the "Rise of the Machines" (sorry, Ahnuld). Machines forced gym goers to work muscles in relative isolation, "relative" because you can't "isolate" one muscle and make it work without having others work as well. Gym owners of the machine age also discovered they could crank a lot of people through a gym in a minimal amount of time with minimal supervision and training. They no longer needed to hire a bunch of trainers, nor had to spend more than one session teaching clients how to use the machines.

So people got weaker, got more injuries (machines force you to move in unnatural ways) and also didn't get the results they thought they should have. Treadmills, ellipticals and other cardio machines were added because people weren't increasing their heart rates.

In the 1970s, jogging became, and still is, a very popular way to "get in shape," but it too led to more injuries, especially of the ankles, knees, hips and lower back. These injuries were, and are, caused by poor shoes, poor running technique, running on asphalt and concrete, and, in general, running too much. Joggers lost weight but mostly burned muscle, so while they looked thin and fit, in reality they were "skinny fat"—thin but with a high percentage of body fat (mid- to upper 20s or higher). Research from the last ten years or so, including a study done by Elliott, Wagner and Chiu, have shown that long, slow-distance running or steady-state exercise tends to use muscle as fuel instead of fat; since muscle is burned, fat is stored.

In the last 10 to 15 years, "old school" training methods have seen a resurgence. These methods involve full-body functional movements that simultaneously build strength and improve cardiovascular function. Basically, they strive to build good, solid, functional muscle and spend less time doing cardio. Kettlebells are the perfect tool for this. Properly done, all kettlebell exercises involve the core directly. They teach you to use the legs and hips for power development, and improve the strength of connective tissue (ligaments and tendons) as well as muscles. In fact, the kettlebell's offset weight strengthens your body from the inside out, increasing bone density, ligament strength and pliability, tendon strength and muscle density. Kettlebells help improve blood flow to the ligaments, which normally get very little (that's why it takes so long to heal a ligament injury like an ankle sprain), and creates a body that is much more resistant to strains, pulls and tears, unlike isolation weight lifting.

KETTLEBELLS AS SPORT

Among kettlebell users are a group who lift for sport. In the U.S., the sport is known as "GS," which stands for "Girevoy Sport" (*girevoy* is Russian for "weight lifting"). Others refer to it as "kettlebell sport" or "KB sport." Although it's certainly not as popular as soccer or tennis, GS is fairly well-known in Europe and the countries of the former Soviet Union. In the U.S., the sport is slowly gaining recognition and competitions are held all over the country.

There are several categories in GS, the most well-known being the biathlon, which consists of two lifts: the double jerk and the one-arm snatch. The jerk is done first: Competitors jerk two bells from rack to overhead for ten minutes or until the bells lower from rack position, whichever comes first. Since you can't set the bells down, you can rest in the rack position or overhead. Resting in the rack position is brutal: Your chest is loaded with anywhere from 32 kilos (or 70 pounds, the weight of a pair of 16k bells) to 64 kilos (or about 140 pounds, the weight of a pair of 32k bells), depending on your level in the sport. After a minimum 30 minutes of rest, the competitor then competes in the snatch. The snatch portion is also ten minutes long. Competitors are only allowed to switch hands once and cannot set the bell down, therefore they try to go five minutes per hand. The only rest you can get is overhead, which builds very strong traps and deltoids as well as lots of stamina.

Amateurs usually use 24k bells, while those at the Master level (not age related) use a pair of 32k bells for the jerk and one 32k bell for the snatch. The highest level you can reach is Master of Sport, which requires years of dedicated practice to develop the strength, endurance and mental toughness necessary to attain the status.

The other competition in GS is called the Long Cycle, or LCCJ. This is a clean and jerk with two bells, performed in a time frame of ten minutes. The LCCJ requires superb mental toughness as well as physical strength and endurance. It sounds easier because you get a slight break as you re-clean the bells after each jerk, but after nine minutes, you still want to give up.

The LCCJ is trained separately from the biathlon lifts, and most people do LCCJ and biathlon competitions six months apart. In either competition, women are only allowed to use one bell because attempting rack position with two bells can affect breast tissue.

Benefits of Kettlebell Training

Kettlebells are a great tool for building all aspects of fitness. They'll help you build strong muscles and bones and improve your cardio in 20 minutes a day. You won't have to spend an hour a day on a treadmill or a stationary bike—just break out a kettlebell, do some swings, squats and snatches and you'll be amazed at the results you'll get in just four to six weeks of consistent training. It's fairly easy to integrate kettlebell training into an existing workout. No matter what your fitness goals are or whether you're training for a triathlon or an MMA match, adding some kettlebell exercises will make you stronger and improve your endurance and core strength.

Kettlebell training will:

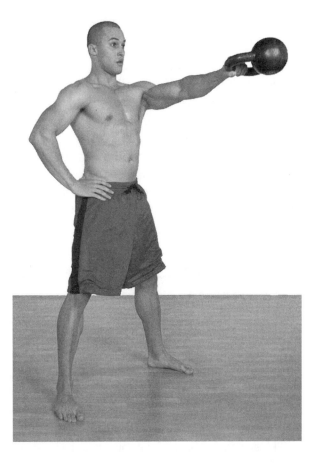

- **Improve strength:** The stronger you are now, the stronger you'll be when you get older.

- **Improve bone density:** As with strength, the more bone density you have now, the more you'll have when you're 80.

- **Improve your balance and coordination:** I'm a strong advocate for training on one leg as much as possible to improve your balance, ankle strength and knee stability; doing so also hits the core hard. When you walk, only one foot is on the ground at any one time, likewise when you run. It makes sense to train on one foot when possible.

- **Increase cardio function:** You'll get your cardio and strength training in one workout. No more doing an hour of weights and another hour on a boring cardio machine.

- **Improve focus.**

- **Teach your body new ways to move.**

- **Teach your body how to recruit the entire body instead of isolating one area.**

Before You Begin

Although this book is set up in a way I feel will let anyone safely and effectively learn kettlebells, it's a good idea to get clearance from your health care provider if you have any health issues or haven't trained hard in over six months. Also get checked out if you're over 40 or pregnant. Use common sense!

While kettlebell exercises may look easy, there are a lot of technical details in all the exercises. I've tried to be as clear and precise as I can be in text, but some people may still have a hard time figuring out if they're moving

the right way. I often have new clients say they learned their kettlebell techniques from a video or book and are now experiencing back problems. It's always caused by incorrect form, and incorrect form almost always leads to injury.

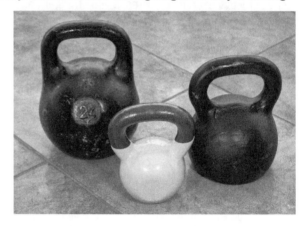

For this reason, you may want to take a few lessons with a qualified kettlebell instructor to make sure you're doing everything correctly. You probably wouldn't try to learn a martial art or play golf from just a book or video, would you? You'd want someone with an expert eye to teach you proper technique and fix the little things that make a huge difference in your game. The same thing goes for kettlebells. For a list of top-quality certifying bodies, visit iron-body.com/certifications. Once you get a feel for the basic movements, you can use this book to enhance your workouts.

CHOOSING THE RIGHT KETTLEBELL

If you're serious about kettlebell training, you'll need to invest in several of them. One is usually not enough. If you pick a weight you can press overhead, it'll be too light for lower body work. If you pick one heavy enough for squats and other lower body work, it's probably going to be too heavy to press overhead.

Typically I recommend three bells: one for pressing; one for lower-body work; and one for swings, cleans and some of the other more dynamic exercises. For **pressing**, men usually need a 16k/35lb bell while women need a 6k/13lb or 8k/17lb bell. If you're used to pressing, you may choose a heavier bell. For **lower-body** work such as 1-leg deadlifts or squats, men typically use a 32k/70lb or 40k/88lb bell while women use a 12k/26lb or 16k/35lb bell. For the *more **dynamic** exercises*, you'll need an in-between size: If your light bell is 16k and heavy is 32k, then get a 24k or 28k; if your heavy bell is a 16k, get a 12k or 14k. Down the road you can purchase twins for your existing bells so that you can start working with two bells at once (doubles), which will take your training to even higher levels.

Kettlebell Styles

There are a lot of kettlebell manufacturers out there, which means there are countless styles to choose from. Some add coatings to the bell that can (negatively) affect the way it moves through your hand. Others have even changed the overall shape, making "loadable" kettlebells where you take the handle and add weight plates to it.

Some bells now have a very small base, which means they tip over more easily. This can make Renegade Rows, and other exercises where the bell supports your weight on the floor, potentially dangerous.

The problem with most "newer" bells is that they don't feel right. Kettlebells weren't designed for two-handed use, so you shouldn't be able to get both hands with all fingers in the handle. However, if the handle diameter is too small, it'll be harder to hold onto. A handle that's too far away from the body of the bell or is too thick will also affect how the bell moves through the hand and where it rests against the arm in rack, overhead or any other lift in which the bell is on the back of the forearm.

The bells I use have a handle that comes straight up or opens up slightly as it comes up from the round part of the bell. I get my bells from the following manufacturers, in no particular order: LifeLineUSA.com, MuscleDriver .com, and WorldKettlebellClub.com. The WKC sells competition steel bells where all the bells are the same dimensions regardless of weight: An 8k bell is the exact same size as a 40k bell, but the 8k is mostly hollow while the 40k is mostly solid. By keeping the size the same, a competitor only has to deal with the change in weight. A dimensional change will cause a change in movement pattern, which means re-grooving the technique.

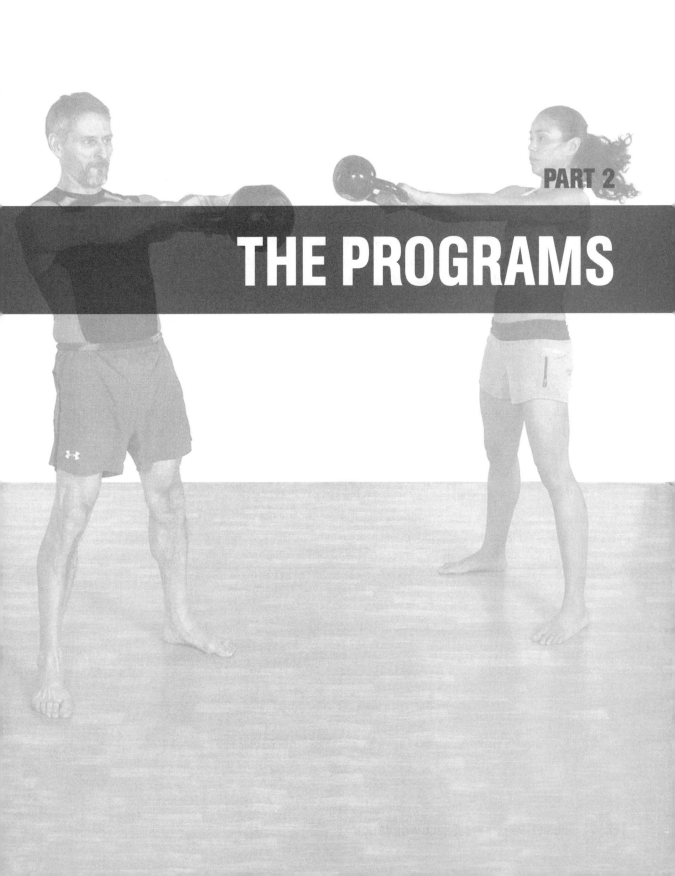

THE PROGRAMS

PART 2

How to Use This Book

This section features several basic workouts for you to follow based on your skill and conditioning level. You'll find detailed, step-by-step instructions for all the exercises in Part 3. The steps to properly perform each exercise are refined from my nearly ten years as a kettlebell instructor. Make sure to read the instructions carefully to attain proper form.

The exercises in Part 3 are presented in a progression, so before you jump into the workouts, you might want to learn the simpler parts of a movement first. Once you can combine them smoothly and fluidly, you can work on the next step of the progression. For example, the basic lift of the swing starts by first learning the Sumo Deadlift, then moves to the 2-Hand Swing. Once you have the 2-Hand Swing down, you'll work with the 1-Hand Swing. You can then move into intermediate-level swings such as the Hand-to-Hand (H2H) Swing and finally the High Pull. However, note that not all lifts have progression/regressions.

> ## TRAIN SAFE
> Don't jump to the advanced lifts (pages 82–109) until you've been training with bells consistently for at least a month and have a very good grasp of the basic lifts.

If you just started working with kettlebells, you're a **beginner**, regardless of your conditioning level. It's very important to keep to the basics for at least three months. You need to practice the kettlebell exercises until they're correct. As with any type of physical activity, you can get hurt using improper technique, going too heavy too soon or losing focus. Dropping a kettlebell on your head or foot is not an option. In fact, we call most of the kettlebell exercises self-correcting: If you mess up and get hurt once, you'll never make that mistake again.

Once you've been working with kettlebells for three months or so, sometimes more, you should be at the **intermediate** level. At this point, you don't have any issues stabilizing your shoulder doing basic lifts. You have near-perfect form in all the swing variations including the high pull, and the clean is smooth.

You're **advanced** if you can handle snatches, jerks, Turkish Getups and Double Windmills with near-perfect form every rep, even when fatigued. Once you've reached the intermediate level, your conditioning plays a bigger part, even more so in the advanced levels. You must be able to perform the more technically challenging lifts while fatigued.

Designing Your Own Program

Most fitness books feed you workouts or programs that last a few months and then you're left on your own or have to buy another book for more programs. I'm going to show you how to develop your own programs and workouts, whether you integrate kettlebell training into an existing workout or train strictly with kettlebells.

The first step is to define your goal. Do you want to drop ten pounds of fat and gain five pounds of muscle? Are you striving to lift a specific weight? Are you competing in kettlebell sport or preparing for a martial arts tournament? Once you pick a goal (two at most), focus on it for two to three months then move on to another goal. This is your program.

In other words, creating a workout is easy but developing a program is much tougher. A workout is done once and can be written with nothing else in mind except working out. A program is, or should be, a series of workouts designed to help you reach a specific goal. Your goal determines the programming. The workouts can be repeated or you may never do the same workout twice in a program.

If your goal is to lose fat or improve conditioning, then you'll need to focus on high-intensity intervals. If you're trying to get stronger, you'll need to do lots of sets with a few reps. If you're trying to build bigger muscles, you'll need to do fewer sets with more reps (in the six to eight range).

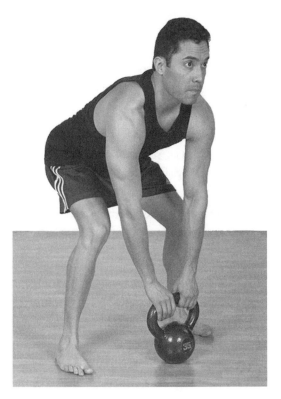

Keep in mind that a workout done as a timed interval is dramatically different than the same workout done for sets and reps. Remember that longer time intervals require lighter weight, and thus more reps (or *volume*), while shorter intervals call for heavier weights (this is considered *intensity*). The same holds true when doing set/rep work. More reps require lighter weights (more volume), while fewer reps and more sets call for heavier weights (more intensity). (For definitions and examples of these various training terms, turn to page 19.)

Follow the K.I.S.S. principle: Keep it simple, stupid. Stick to the basics—a program and the workouts in it don't have to be wild, elaborate things. If you write programs that have a bunch of exercises in them that you don't do well or hate doing, you'll probably skip the workouts that contain those things you hate. On the other hand, doing only exercises you love will create an unbalanced body in many cases. For example, if you hate squats and neglect quad work and focus mostly on hamstring/glute work, you'll end up with hip, knee and back issues because the hamstrings and glutes will overpower the quads.

When creating an actual workout, I try to keep the workout's Rate of Perceived Technique (RPT) at 8 or higher (see page 21 on how to determine how hard you're working). I typically structure a workout like this:

- Joint mobility
- Foam rolling (myofascial release)
- Bodyweight warm-up
- Conditioning
- Strength and skill practice
- Cool-down (stretching, yoga)

You don't need to—and shouldn't—do passive stretching before a workout. Let the movements be your warm-up. By starting with joint mobility, we get things moving a bit. We then move into a more dynamic set (the bodyweight warm-up), where the goal is to raise the heart rate. This is supposed to be moderate work (RPE of 3–5). Take your time and work on improving your movement skills. Note that some fitness pros prefer bodyweight warm-ups before joint mobility.

Next we focus on strength and power, lifting heavier. This is also the time to practice your technique (making sure your form is good) and try new exercises in a controlled fashion. If you're fatigued when learning new skills, you won't be able to keep good form. You can use intervals, ladders, or straight sets and reps. Working supersets is the best way to optimize the work-to-rest ratio and keep the length of the actual workout to 25 to 30 minutes. You may have noticed a lack of "ab" work in this book. That's because everything you do with kettlebells—including heavy deadlifts, rows, swings and jerks—is core work. In crafting your programs and workouts, add in some heavy Low Windmills for oblique work and heavy Goblet or Front Squats to target your rectus abdominis (otherwise known as the six-pack muscles).

For conditioning, we kick things up a notch by going a little lighter and working on short, timed intervals with little to no rest in between. These raise your heart rate and also work on your endurance and mental toughness. Now is the time to go all out but not to the point that your form goes out the window!

After the conditioning section, it's time to cool down your body. Stretching will help keep you moving smoothly and freely and reduce stiffness the next day.

The individual workouts can be varied or you can repeat them if you choose. If you decide to do a different workout each day in your

AVOIDING OVERUSE INJURIES

Since most people spend much of the day at a computer or driving, you should focus more on upper back work than chest work. Typically, you should do twice as much upper back pulling as you do chest pushing.

Most people also tend to be quadriceps dominant, so perform about twice as much glute/hamstring work as you do quad-based work.

program, make sure each one still works on your goal. If you choose to do the same workout several times, you should design two or three workouts and cycle them so you have a high-intensity-day workout and a strength-day workout, plus your light-activity (RPE 3–5) day. It's possible to also flip them by modifying the weight and go from sets/reps to intervals. In other words, take your strength workout and go lighter, and instead of doing 3x5, do 30-second intervals. Or you can transform your high-intensity-day workout into a strength workout by upping the weight and changing over to sets/reps or a shorter interval, say 20 seconds of work and 40 seconds of rest. I advise raw beginners do two or three workouts of moderate volume and intensity to both get used to exercising and to practice their technique. After those first few workouts, you can start going a bit heavier, a bit more intense or both. You should cycle your workouts so you don't overdo it.

There are countless ways to mix up the workouts. You can combine ladders with timed intervals. For example, you could do 2-Hand Swings for 45 seconds, rest 15 seconds, 2-Hand Swings for 30 seconds, rest 15 seconds,

2-Hand Swings for 20 seconds, etc. Each time through you'd go up in weight. You could also do a ladder for a specific length of time (e.g., a Floor Press for 2 minutes) but down as a ladder. That would be 5 presses per arm, then 4 per arm, 3, 2, 1. If you finish before the 2 minutes is up, start over.

When doing interval training, I try to keep the rest interval half the work interval—so a 30-second set of 2-Hand Swings would have a 15-second rest. Unilateral exercises such as the Overhead Press get no rest between arms—you'd press 30 seconds on the right, 30 seconds on the left THEN get a 15-second break before moving on to the next exercise.

For snatches, swings and jerks, the working time frame is typically longer than on other lifts mostly due to the momentum involved in those lifts. A typical interval of snatches would be at least 1 minute per arm, but is usually even longer. In competition, the set is 10 minutes long, you can only switch hands once and you cannot set the bell down. It takes time to build up to that. Intermediate-level kettlebellers should work in the 3–5 minute range for quite some time. Jerks are similarly performed for 10 minutes but are usually done as doubles (using two bells at once). These are brutal if done for 10 minutes. You can't set them down—the only place to get a break is holding them in rack position or overhead. A typical swing set for my clients is usually 2 minutes, but to keep it interesting we break it down like this: 30 seconds 2-Hand Swings, 30 seconds 1-Hand Swings right, 30 seconds 1-Hand Swings left, 30 seconds H2H swings.

To recap:

- Pick a goal.
- Determine the program style (4x7, 3 days per week, 7x4 or something else—see page 22).
- Create workouts that take you to your goal.
- DO THE WORKOUTS!

TERMINOLOGY

The following are some common terms you'll come across in this book and when designing your own programs.

Intensity   Many people think intensity is how hard you're breathing during a workout or how close you are to lying on the floor half dead at the end. In weight lifting circles, however, "intensity" means how *heavy* you lifted, while "volume" refers to how *much* you lifted in terms of reps but the weight is lighter. Heavy is usually 80–100% of your 1 rep max (RM); volume is typically 50–80% of 1RM. The most weight you can lift once on any given exercise at that particular time is 1RM. The number varies based on fatigue and other factors, both physical and mental.

Sets and reps   A set is a series of repetitions (reps) done in a group with no rest. It's usually written out as sets x reps (e.g., 3x5 is 3 sets of 5 reps: You do 5 reps of a Suitcase Deadlift, rest briefly, then repeat 2 more times for a total of 15 reps). Unlike the ladder method (see below), you tend to take a little more rest and ramp up the weight as you go. For example, you might use a 24k bell for the first set of 5, rest for 30 seconds, go up to 28k for set 2, etc., until you reach the total number of sets. It can be tougher to max out on weight when doing sets and reps because you have to be able to do 5 reps of a lift with a given weight.

When working with sets and reps, this generally accepted rule allows you to determine whether you're lifting for strength, power or conditioning:

- *Strength* = many sets and low reps (e.g., 5 sets of 3, or 5x3, using 80–100% 1RM)

- *Power* = fewer sets with a few more reps (e.g., 4x6 or 4x8 using 70–90% 1RM)

- *Hypertrophy (creating big muscles)* = more sets and more reps but less weight (e.g., 8x8, 8x10, 10x10 with 60–70% 1RM)

- *Conditioning* = a few sets of high reps with light to moderate weight (typically 15 reps or more), although many times it's preferable to do conditioning for time rather than sets/reps. You'd try to get as many reps in 30 seconds as possible.

Ladders   Ladders are a version of sets and reps where you increase or decrease the number of reps with each set. On paper, an ascending ladder looks like this: 1/2/3/4/5. There are 5 rungs: For the first rung, or set, you do 1 rep, then 2 reps on the second rung, 3 reps on the third rung, etc. In total, you'll have done 15 reps. You can also do a descending ladder, or 5/4/3/2/1. You'll still do 15 reps but they'll affect your body differently.

Ladders are a great way to build strength and endurance depending on the exercise you use, how heavy and how many rungs. As with sets/reps and timed intervals, the more rungs you have, the lighter the weight you use. One cool thing with ladders is that you can adjust the weight based on where you are on the ladder. When going up a ladder, you can generally use a heavier weight for the first two rungs, then you'll have to drop down in weight. When doing a descending ladder, you fatigue your muscles more quickly so you might not be able to go as heavy on the last two rungs as you did on the first and second rungs of an ascending ladder. Typical rest on either a descending or ascending ladder is usually one controlled breath per rung. This controlled rest also makes it harder to recover on the last few rungs of a descending ladder, further contributing to the lack of power to go max weight.

Intervals   Intervals are timed sets in which you do as many reps as possible in a given time. The longer the interval, the lighter the weight and vice versa. Typically an interval will be written "2-Hand Swing 30s." An average interval is 30 seconds; you'll typically use a lighter bell when going longer and a heavier bell when going shorter.

Supersets   Supersets are simply two exercises done back to back. The exercises should focus on different areas of the body, such as presses and rows. A superset can be done for time or for sets/reps, e.g., "1a Press 5x5 r/l, 1b Row 5x5 r/l" or "1a Press 30s r/l, 1b Row 30s r/l." In the first case, you'd do 5 presses per arm, then immediately do 5 rows per arm for a total of 5 sets. In the second case, you'd do 30 seconds of presses per arm then immediately do 30 seconds of rows per arm, then back to presses. The number of times through is typically also time-based, usually 3 minutes, alternating between the two exercises.

Tri-sets   Tri-sets are the same as supersets except you do three exercises instead of two.

> ## BALANCED TRAINING
>
> For exercises you perform with one hand or one leg, you typically see reps written as r/l or "10/10"—so if you see "5x10/10" or "5x10 r/l," do 5 sets of 10 rows on each arm.
>
> In ladder format, it's assumed you're doing both sides based on the exercise, so a 2-Hand Swing would be done once whereas a 1-Hand Swing would be done twice, once on each side. So "1-Hand Swing 5/4/3/2/1" would be done 5 on the right, 5 on the left then rest; 4 on the right, 4 on the left then rest; down to 1 right, 1 left.

DETERMINING HOW HARD YOU'RE WORKING

We discussed intensity and volume as indicators of how heavy or how much. These terms make it hard to determine how hard you worked, which is relative. If we look at how hard you work and label it Exertion, then examine your Technique in relation to Exertion and finally look at the level of Discomfort (meaning tweaks or strains, things that didn't feel right) and rank those three measures, we get Rate of Perceived Exertion (RPE), Rate of Perceived Technique (RPT) and Rate of Perceived Discomfort (RPD). We'll use a 1–10 scale for all of these.

An RPE of 10 signifies the most extreme, hardest workout you've ever done (you'll never hit a 10). An RPE of 8–9 is very hard (you'll be huffing and puffing and glad you're done; you won't want to do anymore). An RPE of 5–7 is moderate (a good, tough workout that doesn't leave you trashed). An RPE of 3–5 is light, for example some moderate yoga or other easy work. An RPE of 1–3 is an easy walk, tai chi, and joint mobility.

RPT is a relative measure of how well you thought your technique was. This can be done as an average across the entire workout or you can use it for each exercise. You always want to reach for a 10, that being perfect technique, but you'll never get it. Consistently hitting an 8–9 across the board indicates mastery of the various movements, 5–7 means you need more practice (you're at an intermediate skill level), and anything under a 5 means you really need to step back and have someone help you refine your technique.

RPD assesses the amount of discomfort you felt during the workout. This doesn't mean you were uncomfortable because you were sweating or breathing hard, unless you have asthma. This means there was some pain associated with any movement. RPD can and should be applied to the entire workout, from joint mobility to warm-ups

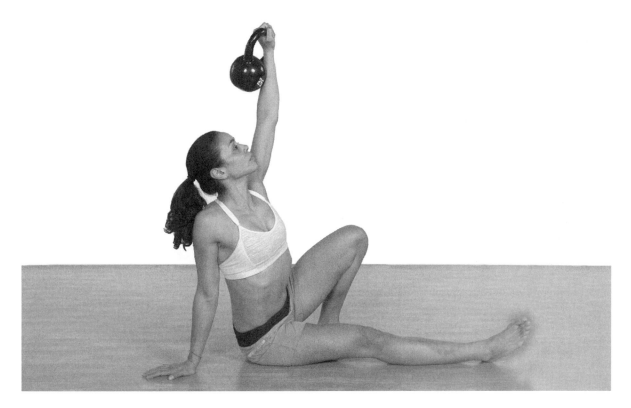

to cool-downs. Anything over a 3 (with 10 being the worst pain you've ever felt) means you need to back off the movement until the RPD is below 3 or stop doing the movement.

Using these three measures, we can now define whether a workout is moderate or intense and, within that context, whether your level of technique held up under the high levels of exertion on high-intensity days. I've found that going more than 30 minutes for high-intensity workouts is counterproductive and can cause injury due to bad form caused by fatigue. If you go hard enough, 20 minutes (not counting warm-ups and cool-downs) is all you really need.

I prefer the cycles that Scott Sonnon has come up with: the 4x7, 7x4 and 3 days per week approach. Choose the one that best meets your lifestyle. (For more info on 4x7, get Sonnon's "4x7 Magic in the Mundane" online from www.rmaxinternational.com.)

The 4x7 looks like this—use a 28-day cycle and start over every fifth day:

Day 1   *No intensity*   RPE 1–3, RPT 8–9, RPD 0 [e.g., joint mobility, tai chi or other restorative practices, but not yoga]

Day 2   *Low*   RPE 3–5, RPT 8–9, RPD 1–3 [e.g., yoga, swim, jog, bike]

Day 3   *Moderate*   RPE 6–8, RPT 8–9, RPD 1–3 [strength day—go heavy with low volume]

Day 4   *High*   RPE 8–9, RPT 8–9, RPD 1–3 [high volume, high energy]

I tend to make my Moderate day a strength-based workout and my High day all-out conditioning.

The 7x4 flips the 4x7 and looks like this:

Days 1–2   *No intensity*   RPE 1–3

Days 3–4   *Low*   RPE 3–5

Days 5–6   *Moderate*   RPE 5–7

Day 7   *High*   RPE 8+

The 3x7 program cycles like this:

Day 1   *Moderate intensity*   RPE 5–7

Day 2   *No*   RPE 1–3

Day 3   *High*   RPE 8+

Day 4   *Low*   RPE 3–5

Day 5   *High*   RPE 8+

Day 6   *No*   RPE 1–3

Day 7   *Low*   RPE 3–5

Choose one of these and stick with it.

INTEGRATING KETTLEBELLS INTO YOUR EXISTING ROUTINE

As you've seen, there are numerous exercises that can be done with kettlebells, and it can be a bit overwhelming trying to figure out how to incorporate them into an existing workout. Fully incorporating kettlebells into your current program has to be tailored to your specific needs, so it's hard for me to tell you exactly what to do. What I can tell you, however, is: Focus on kettlebell exercises that give you the most bang for the buck based on your goals. Keep it simple, don't get wrapped up in stylistic differences and just do the work!

The easiest way is to tack on a few exercises that complement your goals to the end of an existing program. If you're training in BJJ or MMA and most of your training is matwork or boxing, add in some Turkish Getups and 2-Hand Swings after your skills training. Instead of jumping rope, do high pulls.

If you do traditional bodybuilding, use kettlebell rows instead of dumbbell rows, kettlebell overhead presses instead of dumbbells. Then after the main workout, instead of hitting the treadmill or elliptical machine, do high pulls for timed sets of 30 seconds per arm for 5 sets. Even better, just do 3 minutes of high pulls with no rest. You could substitute swings instead of high pulls, but you wouldn't get the heart rate up as much as with high pulls. Swings and high pulls will also develop more powerful glutes and hamstrings. Doing timed sets of the clean and jerk is also a great way to improve your endurance and mental toughness. Try doing a 10-minute set with one hand and switch at the 5-minute mark. Don't go heavy! If you do dumbbell bench presses, do kettlebell floor presses instead. Try some heavy Goblet Squats instead of barbell front squats. It may feel light compared to the barbell, but the Goblet Squat should hit the core pretty hard.

If you play golf, add in Windmills to whatever your current program is to strengthen the core. In addition, 1-Leg Deadlifts will help strengthen the obliques, which will improve your rotation. Make sure you train both sides equally and, better still, work your off side a bit more than your dominant side to counter some of the issues that occur in the back and shoulders with frequent golfing.

Powerlifters might want to add in 2-Hand Swings. Use a moderate bell and do a few sets of 20 to get the blood flowing as a warm-up, or go heavy after your main deadlift workout (just to get the extra *oomph* into the hamstrings, glutes and core). Also try some contralateral 1-Leg Deadlifts—you'll really feel it in your glutes the next day, and they'll work your obliques too.

For tri-athletes, you do so much endurance work across all three events, consider adding some strength training at the end of your primary workouts. On bike day, do snatches or jerks after you get in your miles. On running day, do presses (both floor and overhead), then do rows to balance things out. After your swimming day, put in some deadlift variations or squats. Don't go crazy, though—you don't want to impede recovery, so stay on the moderate side in terms of RPE.

Everyone can benefit from doing Turkish Getups—they're just a great overall movement. You work on shoulder stability, mobility and strength as well as body control, awareness and coordination. You'll work just about every muscle in the body as you move up and down off the floor. Doing a few sets with moderate weight is a great way to warm up. However, please don't do them when extremely fatigued—this can be dangerous.

WORKOUT 1: SCALED EXERCISES FOR BEG/INT/ADV

	EXERCISE	REPS/TIME	REST
WARM-UP	Bootstrapper p. 117	45s	15s
	Spiderman Crawl with twist p. 118	45s	15s
	Alternating Forward Prisoner Lunge p. 122	45s	15s
	Side-to-Side Stretch Lunge p. 120	45s	15s
	Halo p. 126	30s r/l	
	Rest 1 minute.		
ROUND 1	2-Hand Swing p. 42	1 min	15s
	Push-Up p. 112	30s	
	Rest 30 seconds.		
ROUND 2	**B & I:** 1-Hand Swing (30s r/l) p. 43 **A:** Double Swing p. 48	1 min	15s
	B & I: Goblet Squat p. 72 **A:** Double Front Squat p. 74	30s	15s
	Bodyweight Row (Renegade Row with no bells) p. 115	30s	
	Rest 30 seconds.		
ROUND 3	**B:** Suitcase Deadlift p. 65 **I:** 1-Leg Suitcase Deadlift p. 66 **A:** Stiff-Legged 1-Leg Deadlift p. 68	30s r/l	15s
	Floor Press p. 75	30s r/l	15s
	Low Plank: Static Hold p. 113	1 min	
	Rest 30 seconds.		

EXERCISE	REPS/TIME	REST
B & I: Row p. 77	30s r/l	15s
A: Renegade Row p. 82	1 min	15s
Front Squat p. 74	30s r/l	15s
Getup Sit-Up p. 101	30s r/l	
Rest 30 seconds.		
B & I: Dead Clean p. 52	30s r/l	15s
A: Double Dead Clean p. 56	1 min	15s
Overhead Press p. 60	30s r/l	15s
Push-Up p. 112	30s	
Rest 30 seconds.		
Hand-to-Hand Swing p. 45	1 min	15s
B: Low Windmill p. 104 **I:** Overhead Windmill p. 105 **A:** Double Windmill p. 106	30s r/l	15s
B: Static Lunge p. 123 **I:** Prisoner Static Lunge p. 123 **A:** "Y" Static Lunge p. 123	30s r/l	
Rest 30 seconds.		
B: 1-Hand Swing p. 43 **I:** High Pull p. 47 **A:** Pendulum Snatch p. 89	30s r/l	15s
B: High Plank on Knees p. 113 **I & A:** High Plank p. 113	1 min	15s
B: Jumping Jacks p. 119 **I:** Jumping Jacks with arm scissor p. 119 **A:** Jumping Jacks with arm swings p. 119	30s	

ROUND 4 · ROUND 5 · ROUND 6 · ROUND 7

WORKOUT 2: BEGINNER GENERAL CONDITIONING

Repeat the 4 rounds starting with Sumo Deadlift for a total of 2 times through.

	EXERCISE	REPS/TIME	REST
WARM-UP	Bootstrapper p. 117	45s	15s
	Spiderman Crawl with twist p. 118	45s	15s
	1-Leg Stiff-Leg Reach p. 125	45s	15s
	Side-to-Side Stepping Lunge p. 121	45s	
	Rest 1 minute.		
ROUND 1	Sumo Deadlift p. 40	30s	15s
	Push-Up p. 112	30s	15s
	Row p. 77	30s r/l	15s
	Bodyweight Squat p. 124	30s	
	Rest 1 minute.		
ROUND 2	2-Hand Swing p. 42	30s	15s
	Middle Plank Static Hold p. 113	30s	15s
	Front Squat p. 74	30s r/l	15s
	Mountain Climber p. 115	30s	
	Rest 1 minute.		
ROUND 3	1-Hand Swing p. 43	30s r/l	15s
	Burpee Level 1 p. 116	30s	15s
	Overhead Press p. 60	30s r/l	15s
	Sit-Through p. 128	30s	
	Rest 1 minute.		

EXERCISE	REPS/TIME	REST
Dead Clean *p. 52*	30s r/l	15s
High Plank: Static Hold *p. 113*	30s	15s
Goblet Squat *p. 72*	30s	15s
Low Windmill *p. 104*	30s r/l	
Rest 1 minute.		

ROUND 4

WORKOUT 3: BEGINNER STRENGTH

	EXERCISE	REPS/TIME	REST
WARM-UP	Bootstrapper p. 117	45s	15s
	Spiderman Crawl with twist p. 118	45s	15s
	Alternating Forward "Y" Lunge p. 122	45s	15s
	Side-to-Side Stepping Lunge p. 121	45s	15s
	Push-Up p. 112	45s	
	Rest 30 seconds.		

Ladder supersets (e.g., do 5 Overhead Presses r/l then 5 Front Squats, 4 Overhead Presses r/l then 4 Front Squats, etc.)

1a) Overhead Press p. 60	5/4/3/2/1 r/l
1b) Front Squat p. 74	5/4/3/2/1 r/l
2a) Row p. 77	5/4/3/2/1 r/l
2b) Floor Press p. 75	5/4/3/2/1 r/l
3a) Low Windmill p. 104	5/4/3/2/1 r/l
3b) Suitcase Deadlift p. 65	5/4/3/2/1 r/l
1a) High Pull p. 47	10/9/8/7/6/5/4/3/2/1 r/l
1b) Burpee Level 1 or 2 p. 116	10/9/8/7/6/5/4/3/2/1

WORKOUT 4: INTERMEDIATE STRENGTH

	EXERCISE	REPS/TIME	REST
WARM-UP	Bootstrapper p. 117	45s	15s
	Spiderman Crawl with twist p. 118	45s	15s
	"Y" Squat p. 124	45s	15s
	Side-to-Side Stepping Lunge p. 121	45s	15s
	Push-Up p. 112	45s	
	Rest 1 minute.		
	Turkish Getup p. 98 (alternate arms each rep)	3x5/5	1–2 min
	Overhead Press p. 60	3x5/5	1 min
	Front Squat p. 74	3x5/5	1 min
	Row p. 77	3x5/5	1 min
	Suitcase Deadlift p. 65	3x5/5	1 min
	Burpee Level 1 or 2 p. 116	20 sec work/10 sec rest for 4 min	

WORKOUT 5: INTERMEDIATE GENERAL CONDITIONING

	EXERCISE	REPS/TIME	REST
WARM-UP	Bootstrapper p. 117	45s	15s
	Spiderman Crawl with twist p. 118	45s	15s
	"Y" Bodyweight Squat p. 124	45s	15s
	Side-to-Side Stepping Lunge p. 121	45s	15s
	Push-Up p. 112	45s	
	Rest 1 minute.		
ROUND 1	2-Hand Swing p. 42	30s	0
	1-Hand Swing R p. 43	30s	0
	1-Hand Swing L p. 43	30s	0
	Hand-to-Hand Swing p. 45	30s	
	Rest 1 minute.		
ROUND 2	Front Squat p. 74	30s r/l	15s
	Dead Clean p. 52	30s r/l	15s
	Overhead Press p. 60	30s r/l	15s
	Row p. 77	30s r/l	15s
	Push-Up p. 112	30s	
	Rest 1 minute; repeat Rounds 1 and 2 a total of 3x.		
ROUND 3	1-Arm Jerk (no rest, 1 hand switch only) p. 108	3 min r/l	

WORKOUT 6: ADVANCED STRENGTH

Do this sequence 3 to 5 times total, with minimal rest between lifts and sets; 5 times will take about an hour.

EXERCISE	REPS/TIME	REST
Renegade Row (alternate arms) p. 82	5 r/l	
Double Dead Clean p. 56	5	
1-Arm Jerk p. 108	5 r/l	
Pendulum Snatch p. 89	3 to 5 reps r/l	MAX effort
Double Swing p. 48	10	
Double Front Squat p. 74	5	

WORKOUT 7: ADVANCED CONDITIONING

Ladder supersets: Do 20 snatches per arm then 20 burpees, 18 snatches per arm, 18 burpees, etc.

EXERCISE	REPS/TIME	REST
1a) Pendulum Snatch Descending Ladder p. 89	20/18/16/14/12/10/8/6/4/2	
1b) Burpee Level 3 Descending Ladder p. 117	20/18/16/14/12/10/8/6/4/2	
Rest 3 minutes.		
1-Arm Jerk* p. 108	3 min r/l	2 min
1-Arm Jerk* p. 108	2 min r/l	1 min
1-Arm Jerk* p. 108	1 min r/l	

* Jerks are done per arm for the allotted time then switch and repeat; there is no rest between arms.

WORKOUT 8: ADVANCED POWER + CONDITIONING

	EXERCISE	REPS/TIME	REST
ROUND 1	Burpee Level 1/Dead Snatch* p. 116/p. 86 Dead Snatch, alternate arms each rep	10 reps (5 per arm)	1 min
	Double 1-Leg Suitcase Deadlift p. 66	5 r/l	30s
	Double Push Press p. 62	5	
	*Perform Round 1 5x; rest 1 minute between rounds.*		
ROUND 2	1-Step Alternating Clean p. 93	30s	30s
	Slingshot (right) p. 78	30s	0
	Figure 8 with a Tap p. 80	30s	0
	Slingshot (left) p. 78	30s	0
	Figure 8 with a Tap p. 80	30s	
	*Perform Round 2 5x; rest 1 minute between rounds.*		

* This is a combo exercise with the bell positioned on the floor between the feet where it would be for a Dead Snatch. Perform a Burpee Level 1 but come to a squat position rather than standing. From the squat position, perform a Dead Snatch then return the bell to the floor. You're in a partial squat at this point. Place your hands on the floor, kick back to a push-up position, return to a squat, then Dead Snatch with the other arm.

WORKOUT 9: STRENGTH—AS HEAVY AS POSSIBLE

Do 5 times with minimal rest between exercises and rounds.

EXERCISE	REPS/TIME
2-Hand Swing *p. 42*	10
B: Push Press *p. 62* **I & A:** 1-Arm Jerk *p. 108*	5 r/l
B: Suitcase Deadlift *p. 65* **I & A:** 1-Leg Suitcase Deadlift *p. 66*	5 r/l
B: Low Windmill *p. 104* **I:** Overhead Windmill *p. 105* **A:** Double Windmill *p. 106*	5 r/l
Dead Clean *p. 52*	5 r/l
Goblet Squat *p. 72*	5

WORKOUT 10: CONDITIONING—ALL LEVELS

	EXERCISE	REPS/TIME	REST
WARM-UP	Bootstrapper p. 117	45s	
	Spiderman Crawl with twist p. 118	45s	
	Side-to-Side Stretch Lunge p. 120	45s	
	Upward/Downward Dog p. 133	45s	
	Halo p. 126	30 r/l	
	Rest 1 minute.		
ROUND 1	2-Hand Swing p. 42	1 min	
	Rest 30 seconds.		
ROUND 2	Dead Clean p. 52	30 r/l	15s
	Overhead Press p. 60	30 r/l	15s
	Perform Round 2 2x; rest 30 seconds after the second time through.		
ROUND 3	Dead Clean & Press* p. 52, 60	30 r/l	
	Rest 30 seconds.		
ROUND 4	Goblet Squat p. 72	30s	15s
	Figure 8 with Tap p. 80	30s	15s
	Low Windmill p. 104	30s r/l	15s
	Perform Round 4 2x; rest 30 seconds after the second time through.		
ROUND 5	**B:** 1-Hand Swing p. 43 **I & A:** Hand-to-Hand Swing p. 45	30s r/l (H2H 1 min)	15s
	Row p. 77	30s r/l	
	Perform Round 5 2x; rest 30 seconds after the second time through.		

*The Dead Clean & Press combines the Dead Clean with the Overhead Press: Once you've cleaned the kettlebell, press it overhead.

EXERCISE	REPS/TIME	REST
ROUND 6		
High Pull p. 47	30s r/l	15s
Mountain Climber p. 115	30s	15s
Perform Round 6 2x; rest 30 seconds after the second time through.		
ROUND 7		
Push-Up p. 112	30s	15s
Static Lunge p. 123	30s r/l	15s
Perform Round 7 2x; rest 30 seconds after the second time through.		
ROUND 8		
2-Hand Swing p. 42	30s	0
1-Hand Swing (right) p. 43	30s	0
1-Hand Swing (left) p. 43	30s	0
Hand-to-Hand Swing p. 45	30s	

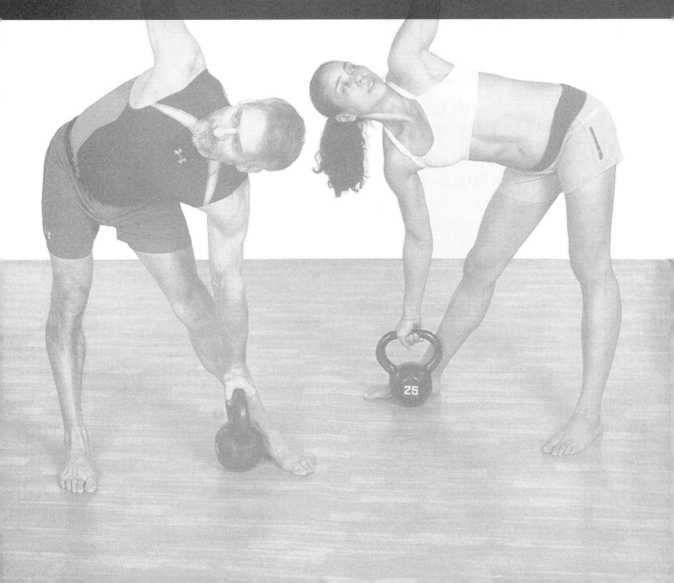

PART 3

THE EXERCISES

Swing Progression

The most basic exercise, the kettlebell swing, is a dynamic movement that primarily involves the hamstrings, glutes and core. However, almost every muscle in the body is activated to some extent when performing the swing. Swinging the kettlebell is about developing power from the rear, sending it through the core and out the arms. It's a ballistic, powerful movement that helps to firm and shape the butt, legs, abs and arms and raise your heart rate quickly, improving your cardiovascular endurance at the same time. You'll no longer need to spend long, boring hours on the treadmill or elliptical—all you need is the swing.

Before we learn the swing, we'll look at a simpler movement that incorporates all the major components of the swing but in a more controlled fashion: the kettlebell *Sumo Deadlift*. Once you have the hip and knee action of this movement down pat, it's time to make it more dynamic and fun (which means harder) with the *2-Hand* and *1-Hand Swings*.

Once you get the hang of the 1-Hand Swing, you can progress to the *Hand-to-Hand (H2H) Swing*. The H2H Swing is a transitional movement: You do a 1-Hand Swing then switch hands in mid-air. There are a couple of reasons for doing the H2H Swing. First, it's used to transition the bell from one arm to the other when doing some other lifts, like the clean or snatch. By being able to smoothly and easily switch hands, you maintain the rhythm of the movement and the breathing. Nothing sucks more than setting the bell down after a hard 30 or 45 seconds of work then starting over on the other side. The H2H Swing allows you to maintain your breathing and pace.

The second reason to practice the H2H Swing is increased core stabilization. With the weight on the side, the opposite obliques have to fire hard to keep you from getting pulled to the side. The abs relax a bit during that the brief period when the bell is at its peak and weightless, but as soon as you grab the bell with the other hand, the opposite obliques fire. You get a continual flow of tension from one side of the body to the other, which makes the core stronger and better able to cope with everyday tasks and athletic endeavors.

Double Swings are another variation, performed the same way as 1-Hand and 2-Hand Swings, but you have a bell in each hand. Aside from that, the main difference is that you have to take a wider stance in order to get the bells between your legs. This wider stance makes it tougher to move the bells because you can't generate as much power when the legs are farther apart.

KEY POINTS FOR ALL SWINGS

- Keep your weight on the mid-part of your foot back to your heels and keep your heels down. If your knees pitch forward, lift your toes.

- You're NOT trying to swing the bell so that it goes higher than your head—there are much better and safer ways to get the bell overhead. Beginners who try to swing a bell above head height tend to lift with their arms but the arms should be passive. Most people bend backward because they can't get their arms overhead with their hands close together. This will cause lower back issues—up to and including disc compression or pinching an already bulging disc—so be careful!

- Don't arch/hyperextend your back to get the bell higher—your back should be flat and vertical.

- Your arms should stay relaxed—they're simply the medium used to transmit the power of the posterior chain (calves, glutes, hamstrings, lower and mid-back) through the torso and into the bell. An overly tight grip will cause your shoulders to rise up by your ears. Keep them down by lifting your chest and pinching your shoulder blades together. Being too tight can also cause elbow tendinitis.

- Keep your elbow "soft." Women especially tend to hyperextend their elbows—keep your elbow relaxed but not limp.

- Don't let your shoulders rise up toward your ears or get pulled forward out of their sockets, especially during a 1-Hand or Hand-to-Hand (H2H) Swing. Keep your shoulder in its socket by pulling your shoulder blade back and down, squeezing your armpit (latissimus dorsi).

HOW HIGH SHOULD IT GO?

The height of the swing is determined only by the power of your hip snap. The bell should float up. The further back (not down) your hips go during the backswing, the higher the bell should go when you bring it back up. However, the bell should not be swung higher than forehead height.

- Pop your hips hard—the hip snap should be very forceful. This will give you strong, tight glutes and thighs.

- Project your energy through the bell and out the bottom, as though you're trying to throw it across the room. The bell is being moved by momentum and hip power, not by lifting with your arms.

- Keep the bell as far away from the floor as you can—*you're not squatting.* Your arms fall and your hips move back to prevent you from getting hit in the groin.

- Keep your wrists straight—if your wrists go up or down, the bell will too. Don't let the bell flop up as it goes behind you.

This precursor to the kettlebell swing is a great exercise in and of itself, especially for building strength.

STARTING POSITION: Stand with your feet a little wider than shoulder width (think of sumo wrestlers) and a bell on the floor between your feet, about even with the balls of your feet. Tighten everything—your abs, glutes and hamstrings. Bend your knees a little and push your hips far back, like you're sitting on a barstool. *Don't squat or bend at the waist;* fold through your hips. Grab the top of the handle with both hands, keeping your weight over the middle and back part of your feet (lift up your toes to check). Keep your chest lifted and look forward.

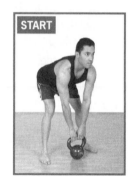

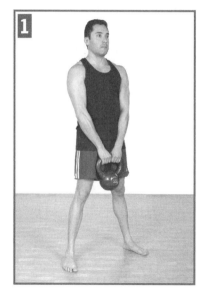

1 Explode with your hips, driving them forward and straightening your knees at the same time. Stand up tall and squeeze your glutes, hamstrings, quads and abs hard. Do not bend backward.

2 Push your hips back and let your knees bend slightly, folding through your hips. The bell returns to the floor between your feet.

Touch the bell to the floor and pick it up again for reps. Do 3 to 5 sets of 10 reps to get the feel.

Things to consider:

- Keeping your chest lifted automatically pulls your shoulder blades back and puts your back in the right position.

- Keep your cervical spine straight—don't bend your neck.

- Let your arms hang straight down from your shoulders—they shouldn't leave the vertical plane. Don't lift with your arms (i.e., don't bend your elbows).

- If you feel this in your back, your upper and lower halves aren't moving together. You may also have used too heavy a bell or squatted down, which typically leads to greater quad and lower back activation.

- If you feel this in your quads any time except when standing erect, you're probably shifting your weight forward to the balls of your feet. Keep your weight on the back part of your foot; lift your toes off the floor if necessary. Your ankles shouldn't move, and your shins stay vertical throughout the movement.

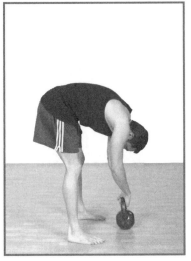

Do not round your back.

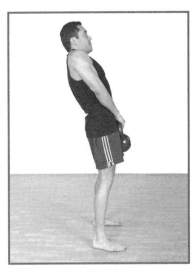

Do not bend backward or shrug your shoulders.

STARTING POSITION: Stand with your feet a little wider than shoulder width, as you did with the Sumo Deadlift (page 40). Place the bell out in front of you so that you have to reach forward a little but still keep your weight on your heels. Push your hips straight back and bend your knees a little.

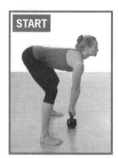
START

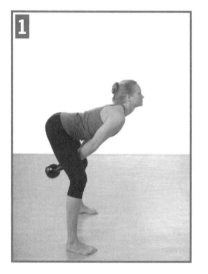
1

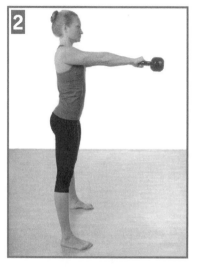
2

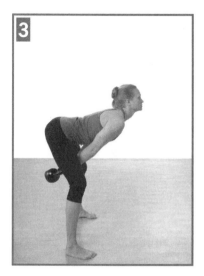
3

1 With both hands on the bell, hike it back between your legs so your forearms are in your groin. Keep your abs tight.

2 Shoot your hips straight forward and drive through your heels. At the same time your hips come forward, your torso rises; your arms and the bell move in an arc forward to approximately chin height (see page 39 on how high it should go). As the bell reaches the peak of the swing, forcefully contract your glutes, hamstrings and abs but keep your arms from the shoulders down "soft"; maintain just enough tension to hold the bell. Your elbows may be *slightly* bent. You should be standing tall with your abs tight and pelvis tucked under. The bottom of the bell is in line with your straight wrists.

3 Reverse the movement by pushing your hips back. The arms trace their path back between your legs. Continue to keep your lats tight, chest out, shoulders down and in, and wrists straight. Think about hiking the bell back behind you as far as you can, not up or down. At this point you should be in the exact same place you were when first starting the swing.

1-HAND SWING

In the 1-Hand Swing, the palm of the working hand should face back and your chest should be square to the front.

STARTING POSITION: Stand with your feet a little wider than shoulder width. Place the bell out in front of you so that you have to reach forward a little, but still keep your weight on your heels. Push your hips straight back and bend your knees a little. Place your free hand on your hip or thigh (see page 44 for other options).

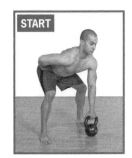

START

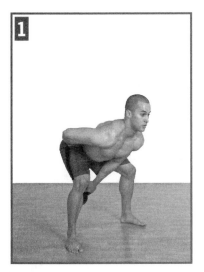

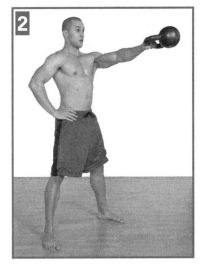

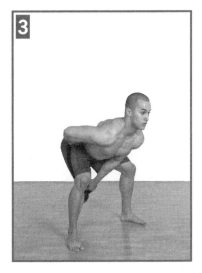

1 With one hand on the bell, hike it back between your legs so your forearm is in your groin. Keep your abs tight.

2 Shoot your hips straight forward and drive through your heels. At the same time your hips come forward, your torso rises; your arms and the bell move in an arc forward to approximately chin height. As the bell reaches the

peak of the swing, forcefully contract your glutes, hamstrings and abs but keep your arm from the shoulders down "soft"; maintain just enough tension to hold the bell. Your elbow may be *slightly* bent. You should be standing tall with your abs tight and pelvis tucked under. The bottom of the bell is in line with your straight wrist.

3 Reverse the movement by pushing your hips back. Continue to keep your lats tight, chest out, shoulders down and in, and wrist straight.

exercise continued on next page

continued from previous page

Other free-hand options

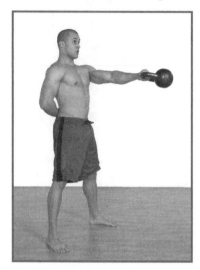

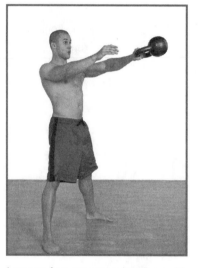

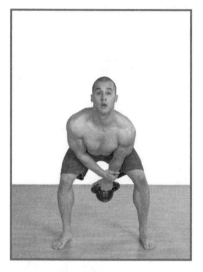

Keep your hand behind your lower back.

Let your free arm move in unison with the working arm.

Place the non-working hand on the wrist of the working arm; this will keep you squared up.

HAND-TO-HAND (H2H) SWING

Make sure you have a good 1-Hand Swing (page 43) before starting on the intermediate-level H2H Swing. It's not as tough as it looks, but it does require some hand-eye coordination and timing. Remember: The H2H is a 1-Hand Swing at all times; you're just exchanging hands at the top of the arc.

STARTING POSITION: Stand with your feet a little wider than shoulder width. Place the bell out in front of you so that you have to reach forward a little, but still keep your weight on your heels. Push your hips straight back and bend your knees a little.

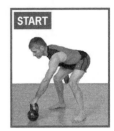
START

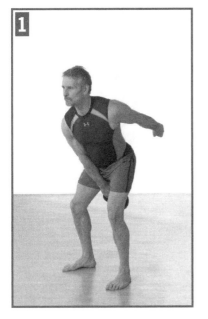

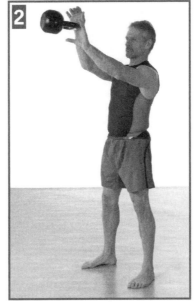

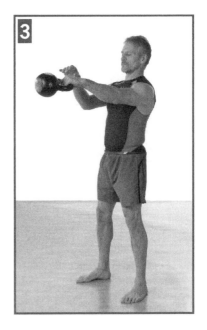

1 Do a 1-Hand Swing (page 43).

2–3 At the point in the swing where the bell is at its highest and just before it starts to drop, slip your free hand over the hand holding the bell and quickly pull the first hand out.

Swing the bell as usual; when it comes back up, switch hands again.

Once you've mastered the basic H2H, you can make it more interesting by letting go of the bell.

STARTING POSITION: Stand with your feet a little wider than shoulder width. Place the bell out in front of you so that you have to reach forward a little, but still keep your weight on your heels. Push your hips straight back and bend your knees a little.

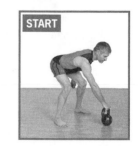

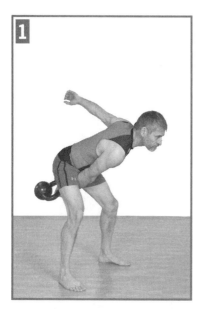

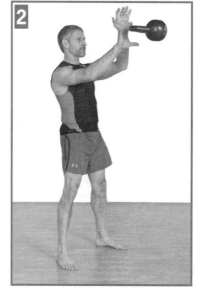

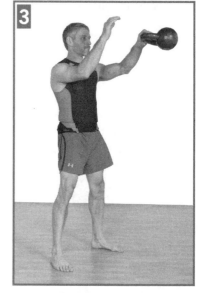

1 Do a 1-Hand Swing (page 43) but let your elbow bend ever so slightly. This will make the bell go up in the air and not out and away from you. This slight elbow bend also prevents you from having to reach out for the bell.

2–3 At the top of the swing, let go of the bell; it should hang for a split second before gravity takes over. Quickly grab the handle with the other hand and continue the swing.

Here's how to tell you're making the switch at the right time:

• *The bell shouldn't flop when you let go of it or grab it. If the bottom of the bell goes up when you switch, you let go too soon. If the bottom drops when you switch, the bell was already moving downward before the switch.*

• *There should be no jerk of the shoulder, elbow or wrist. Any jerking means your timing is off, as described above.*

• *If you feel like your shoulder is being pulled out of its socket or you feel that you're being pulled forward, you didn't bend your elbow. Swinging with a straight elbow will cause the bell to fly out and away from you; if you let go, you'll have to reach out to switch, which will pull you off balance.*

This intermediate-to-advanced-level movement can be looked at as both a hybrid swing and a precursor to the snatch (page 83). In a High Pull, the glutes lock out when the scapula pulls back—not at the top of the swing. This results in a small difference in hip snap timing. Make sure you have very good 1-Hand Swings (page 43) before trying the High Pull.

STARTING POSITION: Perform a 1-Hand Swing.

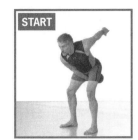

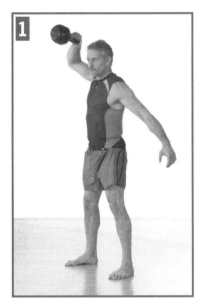

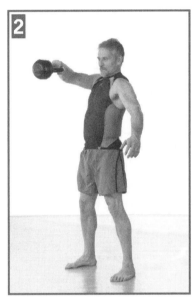

1 As the bell reaches the peak of the swing, retract your scapula. As long as your arm stays relaxed, your elbow will bend as your shoulder goes back. Bring your elbow back to the side of your head until it is bent about 90 degrees. The bell should be in front of and slightly to the outside of your shoulder. Keep it away from your face! Your hips should be locked out at this point. At the top of the High Pull, your forearm should be about parallel to the floor or slightly elevated. Your elbow *must* be higher than your shoulder, and your wrist and forearm should be locked together. If your wrist bends and your hand goes up, the bell will go up too. If you bend your wrist down, the bell will fall.

2 Quickly push the bell back out, letting your arm straighten; your hips should move back just before your elbow straightens out—don't lock your elbow. As your arm straightens, let the bell smoothly resume its normal arc back down between your legs. Remember, this is a swing. Make sure you push your hips *back*, not down, and keep the bell as far from the floor as possible. The bottom of the bell always faces out and away, never up or down, except at the bottom of the swing.

Your form needs to be impeccable on all the easier swing variations before you start working on the Double Swing. Go a little lighter with these: If you usually use a 16k bell for the 1-Hand Swing, you might want to go down to 12k to get the feel of the movement. Swinging a pair of 16k bells feels a *lot* different than doing a 2-Hand Swing with a 32k bell—don't be surprised if you don't swing them nearly as high as the equivalent 2-Hand Swing.

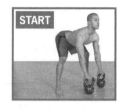

STARTING POSITION: Place two bells of the same weight slightly in front of you. Stand with your feet just wide enough so that the bells can pass through your legs at about knee level (depending on your build, you may need to let the bells pass just below your knees). Try to point your feet straight ahead; if necessary, allow no more than 30 degrees of external rotation. Push your hips back and bend your knees slightly. Grab the handle of a bell in each hand.

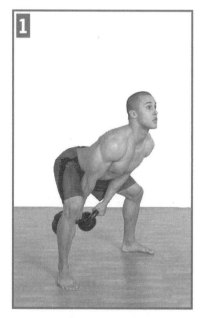

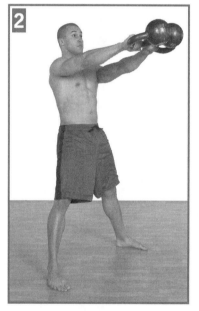

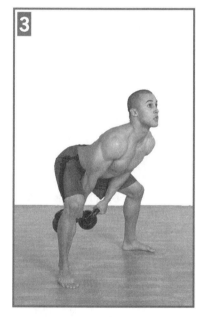

1–2 Hike both bells back between your legs then drive your hips forward, straightening your knees. Pop your hips hard at the end of their range

of motion; keep your abs tight and don't lean back. Don't try to make the bells go higher than they want to go—let your legs do all the work.

3 Hinging through your hips and slightly bending your legs to absorb the bells' energy, let the bells fall back between your legs.

Use your hamstrings and glutes to drive the bells forward again.

Cleans Progression

There are three versions of the single-kettlebell clean: the *Dead Clean*, the *Hang Clean* and the *Pendulum Clean*. These versions plus some others can also be done with two bells. The Dead and Hang Cleans can be learned and practiced without understanding the swing, but I advise you to really work the various swings for a few sessions before working on cleans. Get the feel of the movement; let it become natural.

All three single-bell clean variations involve the same arm movement; the difference is where the clean starts. The most physically demanding of the three, the Dead Clean starts from the floor, or the dead position. Before focusing on Dead Cleans, you may want to practice the 1-Arm Vertical High Pull (page 51) to prevent stress injuries to the elbows and biceps. When doing the Dead Clean, you learn to drop the elbow quickly so that the forearm comes up and learn to move the bell around the forearm to rack position. Most people have trouble getting the bell around the fist to the back of the forearm. To do this, focus on shoving your hand through the handle rather than letting the bell fly over the fist. It's a subtle difference, but doing it right will feel effortless. Doing it wrong will cause lots of bruising on the back of the forearm; you want little to no "air" between the bell and the arm.

The Hang Clean starts with the bell hanging from your arm, elbow straight, between your legs. The rest of the movement is essentially the same as the Dead Clean.

The Pendulum Clean uses a swing-like movement and momentum to move the bell into "rack" position (see page 50). The pendulum action makes it easier to move a kettlebell to rack, but the more-sophisticated movement of this clean is challenging for many people. This clean incorporates the hip snap and movement of the swing but, once the bell is in front of the body, the rest of the movement is just like the Dead and Hang Cleans.

All versions of the clean are technically challenging—there's a lot going on in what looks like a simple movement. It requires full-body power, coordination and timing, and many people struggle to get it down. Typically, you can clean a heavier bell using the swing than you can from the dead position because of momentum. Cleans with a moderate bell feel almost effortless; the catch in the rack position should be smooth, not jarring to the body. You'll know when you're close; it'll feel right.

When practicing cleans, don't overdo it. Less is more. Practice for 10 reps on each arm, then work on something else for a bit, then come back to the clean. If you try too hard, you'll never get it.

Once you're comfortable will the single-bell cleans, there are four variations of the intermediate-level *Double Cleans*: Dead, Hang, Pendulum and Alternating. The first three are done the same way as the single-bell variations, although your stance will be wider to accommodate having both being between the legs.

THE RACK POSITION

The rack position is where the bells wind up after you clean them. It's important to get comfortable in this position since many other movements start from the rack. Without a solid position, your other movements will suffer.

In the position, the bell rests against your forearm, with your elbow tight to your side and into your ribs, and your palm angled toward your body. The bell's handle sits on the bone on the heel of your hand, below your pinky and across to the

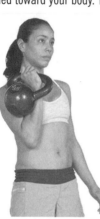

webbing of your thumb/forefinger. The handle of the bell should be at or slightly below your clavicle (collarbone).

Bigger men and some women won't be able to keep this exact position due to their builds. Women will need to keep their arm a little more to the side, and guys may not be able to get their elbow into their ribs, but as long as their triceps are in contact with their ribs at chest height, they should feel solid.

You should not feel the rack position in your shoulders, even with a heavy kettlebell, unless you're holding the rack position for extended periods. The proper position uses the skeletal structure to hold the weight in place. In fact, the hardest part is getting used to breathing with the weight pressing against the chest.

RACK POSITION FOR DOUBLE CLEANS

Start by using the same rack position as when doing singles. Down the road, you'll find there are a couple of different ways to hold the rack depending on the style of lifting you're doing.

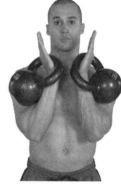

One thing to watch out for: When bringing the bells into rack, it's very easy to catch your fingers between the handles. (Trust me, it hurts!) To prevent smashing your fingers, simply open your hands and point your fingers up as the bells wrap around your forearms. You don't need to keep your hands closed; the bell won't go anywhere.

1-ARM VERTICAL HIGH PULL (1AVHP)

This exercise teaches you the pull on the Dead Clean and how to use the legs to absorb the force of the bell's descent. Practice this movement with a moderate-weight bell until it feels effortless.

STARTING POSITION: Stand with your feet about shoulder-width apart and the bell on the floor between your feet, slightly forward from your instep. Squat down—*don't* bend over—until you can hold the bell in your hand with your elbow straight and your shoulder in its socket.

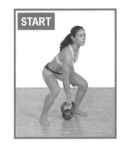

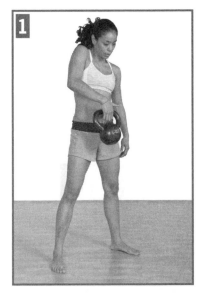

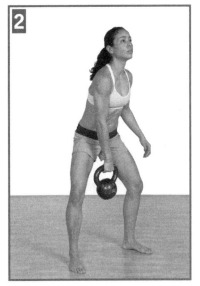

1 Explode up from the squat. Lock your hips, squeeze your glutes and let the momentum raise the bell straight up (don't try to pull the bell; it'll typically end up about waist high). Your shoulder will rise a little and your elbow should have a slight bend—don't force it. If you feel it in your elbow, you're pulling with your arm, not popping from your hips.

2 As soon as the bell stops rising, let it fall back to the floor. Straighten your elbow and squat to match the speed of the falling bell. Don't let the bell slam into the floor (it should just kiss the floor before you drive back up) and don't try to stop it with your arm.

Move up and down quickly, keeping your abs tight and your back upright at all times. Once you've mastered this movement, work on helping the bell float up by lifting your shoulder and allowing your elbow to bend, but don't pull with your arm. The goal is to get the handle of the bell a few inches higher than your navel.

The Dead Clean is the same as the 1AVHP but with more pulling and the bell coming to rest in rack position. The hand orientation is slightly different but the rest of the movement is the same.

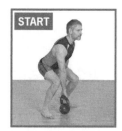

STARTING POSITION: Stand with your feet about shoulder-width apart and the bell on the floor between your feet, angling the handle back toward your left foot. With your right arm hanging straight and your torso upright, squat down and grab the handle so that the webbing between your thumb and forefinger faces your left foot. Look out, not down.

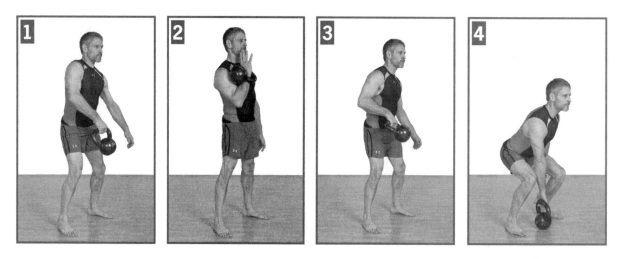

1 Explode through your quads and hips like you're trying to jump straight up. It's OK to come up on the balls of your feet, but don't stay on them. As your legs straighten, keep your arm relaxed; the momentum from the upward hip movement will cause the bell to rise up. As it does, shrug your shoulder a little, with your elbow coming up to about chest height.

2 Now quickly drop your elbow into your ribs and let your forearm and hand come up, shoving your hand through the handle. Keep your thumb pointing toward

your body to allow the bell to wrap around your fist and come to rest on the back of your forearm; keep your wrist straight. The bell's handle should rest across the palm of your hand, diagonally from the base of your pinky to between your thumb and forefinger. You should now be in rack position (page 50).

3 To return the bell to the floor, bump your forearm slightly away from your body to get the bell moving. (As your technique improves, just tip your fingers toward the floor.) Keeping the thumb side

of your hand toward your body, bend your wrist and let the bell fall off the back of your forearm. As the bell falls off your forearm, it also falls from the hip of your hand back into the crook of your fingers. Bend your legs to absorb the force. Keep your arm relaxed but maintain enough tension to hold onto the bell.

4 Squat to place the bell on the floor. Your elbow should be fully straight when the bell touches the floor. Don't slow the bell's descent by muscling it with your arm; it should fall off your forearm.

Things to consider:

- At no time should you feel this in your elbow or biceps. It's not a biceps curl, and the arm is not the prime mover—the legs are. This is primarily a quad exercise.

- If you seem to be pulling with the biceps, remember to "zip your coat," keeping the thumb side of your hand pointing toward your centerline.

- If the bell slams into the back of your forearm, you're either pulling too hard for the weight or getting too much "air" between the bell and your fist. Shove your hand through the handle and keep your arm close to your body.

The only real difference between the Hang Clean and the Dead Clean is that the Hang Clean hangs down between your legs at the start and finish instead of sitting on the floor. The rack position is identical.

STARTING POSITION: Stand with your feet about shoulder-width apart. Hold the handle of the bell in your left hand so that the thumb side of your hand is angled back toward your right leg. Let the bell hang between your legs with your arm straight. Bend your knees and drop your hips a little to do a partial squat.

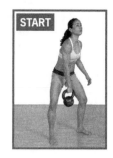

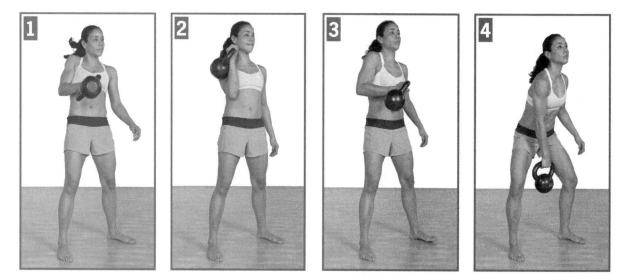

1–2 Drive through your heels and straighten your knees to explode upward. The bell should begin to move upward from the leg drive: Keep your elbow close to your side and shrug your shoulder a little (this should happen naturally). Drop your elbow and let your forearm rise up, shoving your hand through the handle just like with the Dead Clean. You should now be in rack position (page 50).

3–4 To return to starting position, bump your forearm forward a little and bend your wrist, keeping the thumb side of your hand pointed toward your body. As the bell falls off your forearm, it also falls from the hip of your hand back into the crook of your fingers. Straighten your elbow as the bell falls, and bend your legs to absorb the force of the falling bell. Keep your arm relaxed but not loose; maintain enough tension in your arm and hand to hold onto the bell. Don't muscle it down or up—it's all legs.

This variation adds in a new force vector, a rocking movement that can be anything from barely folding at the hips to a nearly full-fledged swing. It's often referred to simply as a "clean."

STARTING POSITION: Stand tall with your feet about shoulder-width apart and hold the bell between your legs at groin height.

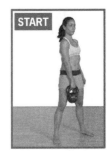
START

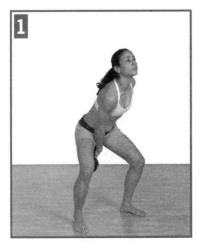
1

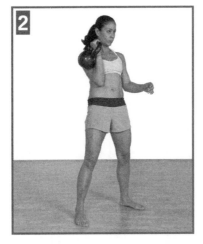
2

3

1 Rock your hips a little and let the bell move forward and backward between your legs.

2 As soon as the bell passes forward through your legs, pull your elbow in tight to your lower ribs and let your forearm rise up.

Keep the thumb side of your hand pointing toward your body. As the bell comes up, shove your hand through the handle. You should now be in rack position (page 50).

3 To dump the bell, bump your forearm forward slightly and let the bell fall off your hand and into your fingers. Straighten your elbow as the bell falls, and bend your knees and push your hips back to let the bell go between your legs.

Things to consider:

• The biggest mistake is trying to do a full swing. Don't let the bell get way out in front of the body. This causes the bell to crash back into you when you try to bring it into rack position. To find the right distance, stand about 2 feet away from a solid wall. If you hit it, the bell is too far out in front. Keep a close, tight arc.

• Don't pull too hard. If you do, the bell winds up smacking the back of your forearm. Because you're using momentum from the hip snap, you don't need as much power to bring the bell to rack. If you can't back off the power, use a heavier bell. (Heavy weight often fixes bad technique.)

• Don't try to tighten up on the handle to keep the bell from banging—keep your grip relaxed during the swing phase and the rack phase. Learn to use the right amount of force for the size bell and clean variation. Squeezing the handle will rip up your hands.

Double Dead Cleans are tough not only because of the increased weight but because your arms move in opposite directions. Your energy and focus are split, as opposed to doing a barbell clean, where both arms are applying force to one object. Start with a pair of light to moderate bells and get the technique down before trying to go heavy.

STARTING POSITION: Stand with both bells on the floor between your feet and grab each bell, just as you did in the one-hand version (page 52). Sink your hips and keep your torso upright.

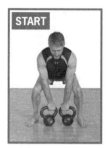

START

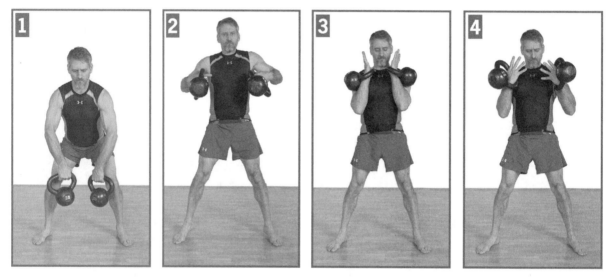

1–2 Driving through your heels, explode straight up. Your shoulders should naturally rise from the hip explosion as the bells come up. Using the upward momentum, let your arms and the bells continue to rise. As the bells reach approximately chest height, drop your elbows and drive your

hands up through the handles. Keep your elbows in close just as you did in the single-arm Dead Clean.

3–4 To put the bells down, bump your elbows a little and bend your wrists so that your fingers point to the floor; let

the bells fall off your forearms into your fingers. As this happens, straighten your arms and sink your hips down, allowing your legs to absorb the force of the bells. The bells should lightly touch the floor. The end position is the same as the start.

DOUBLE HANG CLEAN

These are exactly the same as the single-bell version (page 54), except you're holding two bells and cleaning them at the same time.

STARTING POSITION: Hold a bell in each hand and let them hang between your legs.

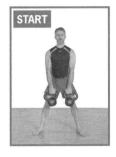
START

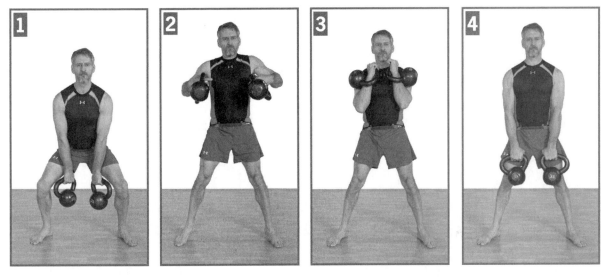

1–2 Bend your knees and explode up, popping your hips.

3 As the bells rise up, drop your elbows quickly into your sides. Watch your fingers! Stand up tall.

4 To return to the hang position, bump your elbows a little and let your wrist bend so that your fingers point to the floor. As the bells fall off your forearms, straighten your arms and bend your knees to sink your body weight. Let your legs—not your arms—catch the weight of the bells.

You need to be able to swing a pair of bells to at least mid-torso or you may not be able to finish this movement without compromising technique. If you feel it in your biceps or shoulders, using your arms too much.

STARTING POSITION: Stand tall and hold the bells between your legs at groin height.

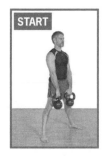
START

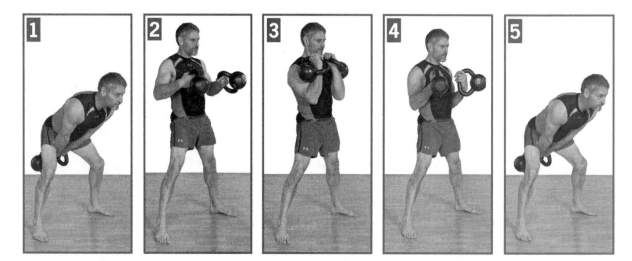

1–2 Just like you did in the Double Swing (page 48), hike the bells behind you then explode forward. As the bells swing forward, keep your upper arms and elbows close to your body.

3 When your hips finish their forward movement, bend your elbows and bring your forearms in, keeping the thumb side of both hands pointed inward. Let the bells wrap around your hands and into rack position; open your hands to keep your fingers from getting smashed. Be careful! Many a finger has been broken by Double Pendulum Cleans!

4–5 Fold your hips back and start to rotate your forearms inward, letting the bells fall into your swing grip as your elbows straighten. Continue to push your hips back—folding, *not* squatting—and keep your upper arms close to your body. Your elbows will straighten completely as the bells start to pass back between your legs.

Overhead Press

The Overhead Press (often called Military Press because it looks as though you're standing at attention) works more than just the shoulders. Done correctly, this traditional strength exercise is a whole-body movement that starts from the ground up. By squeezing every muscle in your body from your toes up to your chest and from your calves to your upper back, you'll create full-body tension that will allow you to lift heavier weights without worrying about getting hurt.

Most people have seen guys in the gym cranking out tons of reps with a light dumbbell at a very fast pace. Doing the press this way tends to work (or overwork, in many cases) the deltoids and the rotator cuff muscles. In order to prevent injury and get the most benefit from the press, move slowly and stay tight. With the Overhead Press, you use the back, instead of the shoulder, to initiate the movement.

There are two lines you can follow when pressing: either straight up, or up, out and in (commonly referred to as the Arnold or Cuban Press). Make sure you can correctly do a Swing or Dead Clean and can hold the bell in proper rack position before working the press.

The *Push Press* is sort of a cheat press. You get to use your legs and hips to get past the "sticking" point you may encounter using a heavy bell in a strict press. The concept is that by getting through the sticking point, you'll get stronger in the rest of the movement, which translates into a stronger press—eventually leading to being able to do a strict press without the cheat. Because the Push Press is more dynamic than the strict press, you'll be moving more quickly and therefore won't be able to generate the same amount of whole-body tension. However, stay as tight as possible.

You can do whichever clean variation (Dead, Hang or Swing) you prefer to get the bell to rack position. I start with the Dead Clean.

STARTING POSITION: Clean the bell and hold it in rack position.

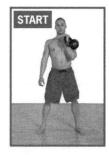

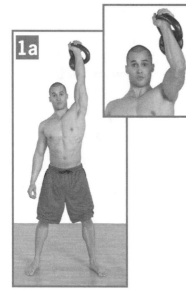

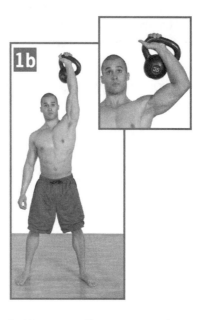

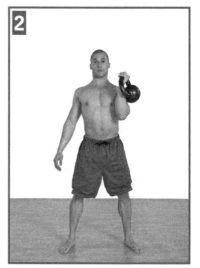

1 Move your feet under your hips and grab the ground with your toes to generate tension from the ground up to your chest, front and back. Squeeze your armpit so your lat touches your triceps. You'll now either:

a. Press the bell straight up by squeezing everything tightly and keeping the movement slow and controlled. Your forearm remains vertical throughout the movement.

b. Move your elbow out toward your side at the same time you start to press. Keep your forearm vertical. When your elbow is nearly straight, your forearm should move up and in. This is the Arnold Press.

For all variations, lock your elbow but make sure your shoulder stays in its socket. Your hand should be directly over your shoulder and your biceps should line up with, but not touch, your ear.

2 Pull the bell back to rack position by reversing the direction of the press. It should feel like you're doing a one-arm pull-up or someone is holding the bell, preventing you from returning it to rack. Make sure you aren't compressing your elbow. Keep your forearm vertical throughout the movement. If it does, you'll begin to feel discomfort in your elbow.

DOUBLE-BELL VARIATION: Clean two bells, using whichever variation (Dead, Hang or Swing) you like. Once they're in rack position, press them both at the same time, using all the tension, breathing and movement patterns you learned on the single press. You can use either the straight line (step 1a) or Arnold Press (step 1b).

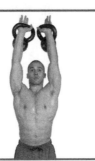

Before trying the Push Press, make sure you can do a clean and a press correctly.

STARTING POSITION: Clean the bell and hold it in rack position.

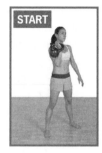

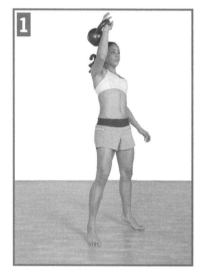

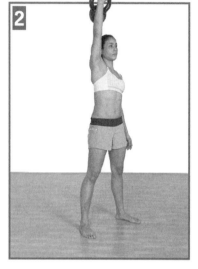

1–2 As you start to push off your lats with your arm for the press, quickly bend your knees slightly and then pop your hips straight up and lock your legs. This little push should help you get the bell up; if not, use more leg drive. Think of throwing the bell up.

3 Bring the bell back to rack.

Things to consider:

• If the bell is just a little too heavy for a strict press, focus on the slow, controlled negative. You should never feel that the bell is out of control.

• If you're truly working on max-weight presses and you're using the Push Press because it's the only way you can get it overhead, you'll have to let the bell drop back into rack rather than doing a negative.

• If you're doing Push Presses as more of a strength/endurance exercise, you'll be moving at a faster pace when both pressing and dropping back to rack (see variation below). It'll be much more fluid and you'll be basically bouncing the bell from rack to overhead and down again.

DOUBLE-BELL VARIATION: This can also be done with two bells.

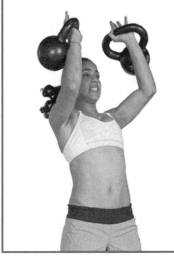

FAST-DROP VARIATION: When the bell is overhead, let it fall straight down. As it does so, come up on your toes a little to meet the bell. As the bell begins to make contact with the front of your shoulder, drop back to a flat-footed position. When your heels contact the floor, the bell should slip back into proper rack position and you should be standing tall, with your glutes and abs tight. To really work on this as a nonstop movement, you'd bend your knees and drive the bell back up instead of ending in rack and restarting the Push Press movement.

Deadlift Progression

The deadlift involves the entire body—the upper back, shoulders, arms and hands are worked just as hard as the hamstrings, glutes, lower back and core. Many times, grip strength is the limiting factor when doing heavy deadlifts with a barbell.

There are several kettlebell deadlift variations (we discussed the Sumo Deadlift in the Swings section on page 40), each working the body in different ways and targeting one part of the body more than another. For example, a 1-Leg Deadlift with one bell hits your core and legs much differently than the same movement performed with a bell in each hand; the second bell helps you balance better on one foot, which means the core doesn't have to fire as hard to keep the torso from rotating. On the other hand, doing a 1-Leg Deadlift with the bell in the hand opposite the standing/working leg tends to make you rotate your body toward the side the bell is on. In order to stay stable and keep your hips and shoulders parallel to the ground, your core has to fire even harder than when the bell is on the same side as the working leg.

KEY POINTS FOR ALL DEADLIFTS

- Go slow and stay tight. One way to control the tempo or speed of the movement is to count in your head (1001, 1002, 1003, 1004, 1005) when moving up and then down.

- Throughout the entire movement, the core should be tight. I make my clients deadlift at a very slow pace. In a 30-second interval they may only get 4 or 5 reps on a side, but they're under full tension for almost the entire time, thereby getting stronger and learning how to stabilize better.

- If you feel yourself being pulled down or losing control of the bell as you place it on the floor, don't go so deep. When you feel yourself start to rotate or otherwise lose form, stop the descent and stand back up. As you get stronger and your range of motion increases, you'll be able to get into the movement more deeply.

- When returning the bell to the floor, don't let your hips shift to the side, don't let your shoulder come out of its socket and don't rotate through the hips or anywhere else in order to reach the floor.

The Suitcase Deadlift gets its name because you start in the same position you would if you were picking up a short suitcase.

STARTING POSITION: Stand with your feet and knees together and place the bell just outside your right foot.

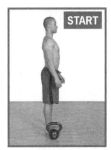

START

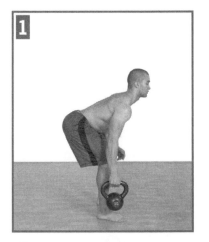

1 Push your hips back and down, letting your knees bend. Keep your weight focused toward the back of your foot (lift your toes if you feel your quads are doing most of the work). This is more like a traditional barbell deadlift than the stiff-legged deadlift that we do during a Swing or Sumo Deadlift. Keeping your torso upright, stick out your chest and look out about 10 feet in front of you, either at a spot on the floor or straight ahead. Don't look straight down or up. Keep your cervical spine aligned with the rest of your spine. Grab the bell's handle.

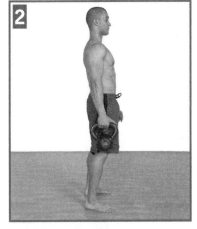

2 Staying very tight and moving at a slow to moderate, controlled pace, drive though your heels and stand up tall, squeezing your glutes, hamstrings, quads and abs at the top.

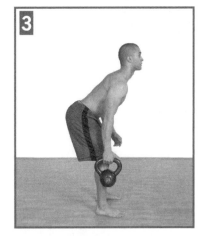

3 Return the bell to the floor by pushing your hips back and down, staying tight. As the bell approaches the floor, make sure your body is still in perfect alignment.

DOUBLE-BELL VARIATION: To do with two bells, just place one bell on the outside of each foot. This version is easier because you have more stability, but it's harder on the glutes and hamstrings because you're generally lifting more weight.

As its name suggests, this intermediate-level deadlift variation is identical to the Suitcase Deadlift (page 65) in terms of hip and knee flexion and torso position. The only difference is that you stand on one leg. If you're going heavy, you should feel your obliques working.

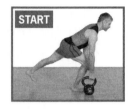

STARTING POSITION: Stand with your feet together and the bell just outside your right toes. Push your hips back and down and grab the handle with your right hand. Keep your chest up and out. Lift your left foot off the ground and straighten it behind you without changing any other part of your position. There should be a straight line between the back of your head and the heel of your foot. Keep your abs tight and your hips locked to prevent your body from rotating; your hips and shoulders must remain parallel to the floor.

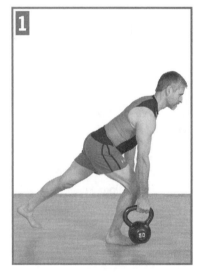

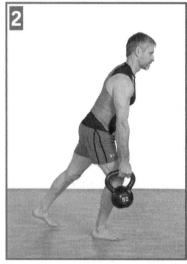

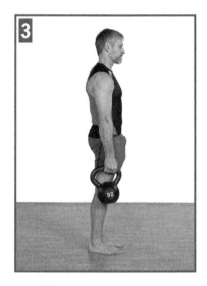

1–3 Drive through your right heel, leading with your shoulders, and push your hips forward. Keep your weight on the back part of your right foot; don't

let it shift toward your toes. As you stand, straighten your right knee and extend your hips. Your left leg should move as a unit with the body; don't let it move indepen-

dently from your hips. Once you're standing tall, you can put the left foot down if you want.

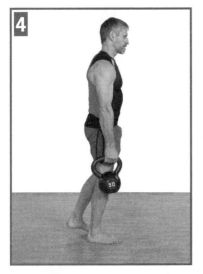

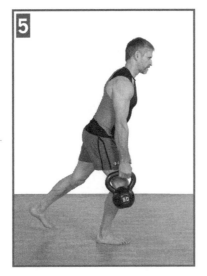

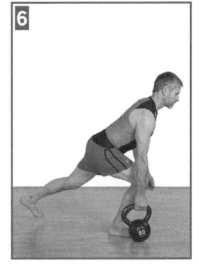

4–6

Return the bell to the floor by pushing your hips back and down in the exact reverse motion of how you stood up. Remember to move your left leg with your body, maintaining a straight line from the back of your head to your heel.

Things to consider:

- When the bell is on the floor, the back foot should be close to the floor with the leg fully extended. The back knee is never bent.

- The hips should never be at the same level or higher than the shoulders. Keep the torso up and the hips down.

- If you twist for balance or your rear leg shifts to one side, your abs and hips aren't firing properly or you're going too heavy. If you're intentionally trying to "max out," this is okay; otherwise, go lighter.

- Keep in control. The bell should never pull you down. If you can't keep control during the descent, go with a lighter bell or stop as soon as you feel the loss of control. If this happens even with a light bell, work on your hamstring and glute flexibility.

- If the knee of the standing leg wobbles as you stand or descend, your glutes may not be firing properly. Use a foam roller on the outside of your hip and thigh, just down to the knee, then try the deadlift again.

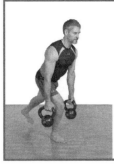

DOUBLE-BELL VARIATION: You can perform this using two bells. Just place the second bell by the outside of the other foot. You should go heavier with two bells.

CONTRA-LATERAL VARIATION: For an extra challenge and more core activation, hold the bell with the hand opposite the working leg (so if you're working your right leg, hold the bell in your left hand).

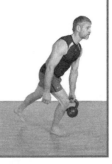

This intermediate-level deadlift variation is the exact same movement as the Sumo Deadlift (page 40) but performed while standing on one foot. Although it's called "stiff-legged," your knee should be slightly bent. This works the lower back a bit more than the suitcase variation. If you're going heavy, you should feel your obliques working.

STARTING POSITION: Stand with your feet together and the bell just outside your right toes.

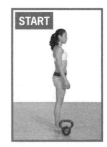

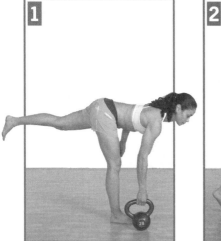 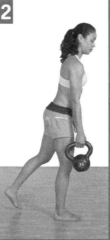 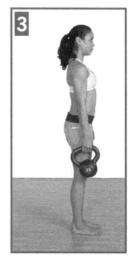 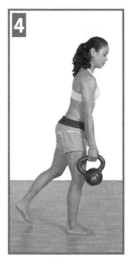

1 Bend your right knee slightly and tip your whole body toward the floor by folding through your hip and letting your left leg come off the floor. Make sure your left leg stays straight and moves with your body. Keep your abs tight and your hips locked to prevent your body from rotating; your hips and shoulders must remain parallel to the floor. Grab the bell's handle with your right hand.

2–3 Squeezing your hamstrings and glutes, drive your hips forward and lift your torso up at the same time to return to standing.

4 Push your hips back, bend your knee slightly and fold through your hip again to return the bell to the floor.

Things to consider:

- Move slowly and take your time. More time under tension (T.U.T.) means better strength and stability and a much stronger core.

- If you find yourself getting pulled down or are losing control of your body as you place the bell on the floor, use a lighter bell or don't go all the way down. Stop at the place where you feel your form break.

DOUBLE-BELL VARIATION: You can perform this using two bells. Just place the second bell by the outside of the other foot. Using two bells takes a lot of the balance issues out of the equation, but because you can—and should—go heavier, it should still be difficult and you should still feel it in your abs.

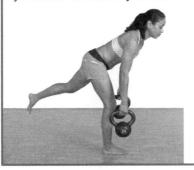

CONTRA-LATERAL VARIATION: For an extra challenge and more core activation, hold the bell with the hand opposite the working leg (so if you're working your right leg, hold the bell in your left hand).

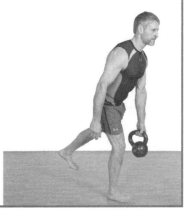

Squat Progression

There are several ways to do squats using kettlebells, and most of them are considered "front" squats (the bell is in front of the body) as opposed to "back" squats (a weight is on the upper back).

The *Sumo Squat* is usually the easiest for people to get the feel for and takes its name from the Japanese sumo wrestler's wide stance. It looks a lot like the Sumo Deadlift (page 40), but in the Sumo Squat the hips go down and back, whereas in the Sumo Deadlift the hips go back and the knees barely bend. The Sumo Squat targets the quads and glutes (if you go deep enough), while the Sumo Deadlift works the hamstrings, glutes and back.

With the *Goblet Squat*, you hold the bell in front of your solar plexus. This makes the abs (specifically the rectus abdominis, or six-pack muscles) work a lot harder; you should really feel them after you've finished your sets. The Goblet Squat, if you go heavy enough or do a lot of reps, is also the only kettlebell exercise that truly works the biceps. They're the primary muscles involved in holding the bell in front of you.

When you do the *Front Squat*, your body will actually move away from your forearm. As you stand, your body will move back into your forearm. Your forearm doesn't move. The Front Squat activates the obliques more because they have to fire harder in order to keep you from falling to one side.

KEY POINTS FOR ALL SQUATS

• Activate your hip flexors—pull yourself down.

• Get your belly between your hips.

• Go as deep as you can but keep your torso upright.

• If your upper body starts to tip forward, stop and go back up. Work on ankle and back flexibility in addition to practicing the squat.

• Keep your feet flat on the floor.

• Keep your weight on the back part of your foot and the outside edge.

• Spread the ground apart with your feet.

• Keep your knees out and in line with your toes.

• Point your feet outward no more than 30 degrees.

• Don't let your hips and butt come up before your shoulders. This is a sign of weak abs and/or the bell being too heavy.

• Keep your head facing forward and look up with your eyes throughout the movement. This will help you stay strong and prevents your hips from coming up before your shoulders.

STARTING POSITION: Stand with your feet a bit wider than shoulder width and the bell between your feet (more toward your toes than your heels). Let your arms hang straight down and squat by pulling your hips down; try to keep your chest up and out. Only go deep enough to grab the handle with both hands, keeping your elbows straight.

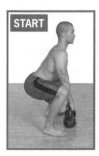

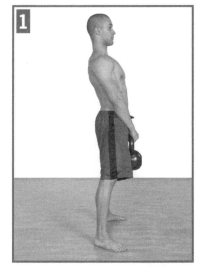

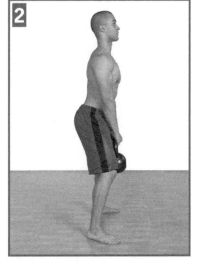

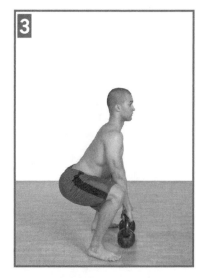

1 Driving through your heels and leading with your shoulders, stand up tall and squeeze your glutes, hamstrings, quads and abs at the top. Don't let your butt come up first.

2–3 To put the bell on the floor, pull your hips down, keeping your torso upright as much possible and your arms straight. Once the bell is on the floor, stop your descent and

reverse to stand back up. Don't let go of the handle until you have completed your reps or the time interval.

DOUBLE-BELL VARIATION: You can also do the Sumo Squat with two bells.

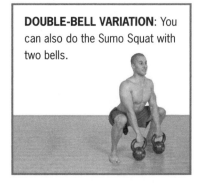

The Goblet Squat is the same movement as the Sumo Squat (page 71), except you hold the bell in front of your solar plexus. Make sure the bell stays in front of your solar plexus; don't let it rest on your body. It should be a few inches in front of you.

STARTING POSITION: Stand with your feet a bit wider than shoulder width. Get the bell into position at your chest (see page 73).

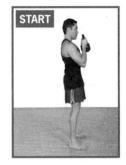

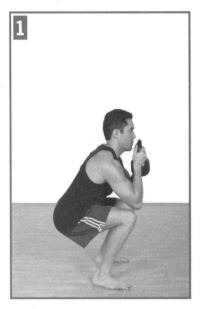

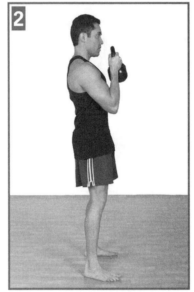

1 Activating your hip flexors and abs, pull yourself down. Try to get your hips below your knees. Regardless of the depth of your squat, keep your torso upright and your weight on your heels.

2 Driving through your heels and leading with your shoulders, stand up tall and squeeze your glutes, hamstrings, quads and abs at the top.

To return the bell to the floor after finishing your set or interval, smoothly let the bell drop toward the floor and allow your hands to slide from the sides of the handle to the top. Your arms will straighten out. At the same time, squat down and gently place the bell on the floor.

VARIATION: One combination you could do is a Sumo Squat then, bringing the bell to Goblet Squat position, a Goblet Squat, and finally a Sumo Squat to put it back on the floor. You can even add in a squat thrust to make it tougher.

GETTING THE BELL INTO POSITION

1 Stand with your feet a bit wider than shoulder width and the bell between your feet (more toward your toes than your heels). Let your arms hang straight down and squat by pulling your hips down; try to keep your chest up and out. Only go deep enough to grab the handle with both hands, keeping your elbows straight.

2–3 Keeping your chest up and back flat, stand up quickly, popping your hips and squeezing your glutes at the top. As you finish the upward hip drive, use your hands to guide the bell up in front of your chest (don't let it rest on your body). As the bell moves up, quickly slide your hands from the tops to the sides of the handles and drop your elbows so that they point down.*

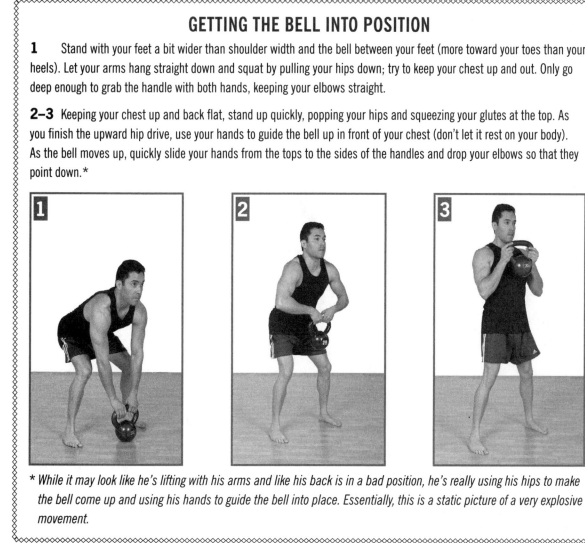

While it may look like he's lifting with his arms and like his back is in a bad position, he's really using his hips to make the bell come up and using his hands to guide the bell into place. Essentially, this is a static picture of a very explosive movement.

Before you can do a Front Squat (sometimes called a "racked" squat), you must know how to rack your bell (see page 50).

STARTING POSITION: Bring the bell to a racked position. Keep your elbow and forearm vertically stationary. Don't lift your elbow up to hold the bell.

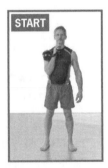

START

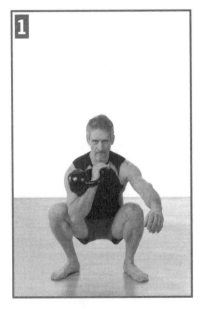

1

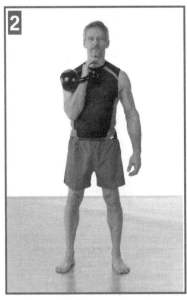

2

1 Keeping your abs tight, pull yourself down. Try to get your belly between your legs and your hips below your knees. Keep your knees aligned with your toes, your weight on your heels and outside edges of your feet; push the ground away from your body and spread it apart with your feet.

2 To return to standing, push your knees apart, lead with your chest and drive from your heels. Your knees and hips move together.

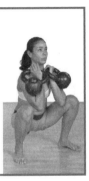

DOUBLE-BELL VARIATION: You can also do this with two bells.

Floor Press

The Floor Press, done lying on the floor and pressing one or two kettlebells up, is a great exercise for developing the pectoralis major and minor. It also works the triceps and some of the muscles of the upper back, such as the latissimus dorsi and serratus anterior. I have my clients focus on pressing from their back, using the lats to drive (similar to a standard overhead press).

The Floor Press can be done with the legs straight or with the knees bent and feet flat on the floor. The first way is preferable as it allows you to keep your lower body tighter. As with all "grinding" movements (slow, deliberate, controlled lifts), we want the entire body to be tight, bracing the abs and squeezing every muscle as much as possible.

FLOOR PRESS

STARTING POSITION: Lie on your back with your legs straight along the floor. (If you feel lower back strain, do the modification below.) Get the bell into position (see page 76).

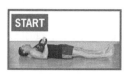

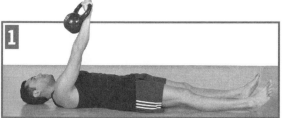

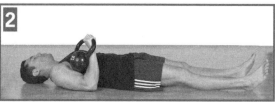

1 Squeeze everything tight and press the bell up, locking your elbow. Don't let your elbow flare out. The inside of your arm should brush your side while pressing up and pulling down. Your forearm and hand should be just below the level of your chest when your arm is fully extended. Don't allow your hand and bell to be over your shoulder or face. This weak position recruits mostly deltoids to press the bell rather than the pecs and lats. We want full-body involvement.

2 Keeping your forearm vertical, pull the bell back to starting position.

MODIFICATION: Bend your knees and place your feet flat on the floor.

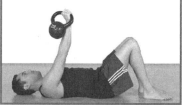

DOUBLE-BELL VARIATION: When doing the Double Floor Press, some people naturally rotate the forearms as they press so the hands wind up pointing toward the feet when the arms are fully extended. That's OK, although I feel it's a slightly weaker position and tends to put a bit more stress on the shoulders. As you bring the bells back down, rotate the forearms back so the palms face each other at the bottom.

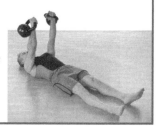

GETTING YOUR BELLS INTO POSITION

Before you can do the Floor Press, you'll need to learn how to get the bell off the floor and into the proper starting position. Whether you use one bell or two, the bell should be positioned in the hand and against the forearm, exactly as it would be if you were holding it in the rack position (see page 50) while standing.

USING ONE BELL:

1 Lie flat on your back with the bell positioned about a foot to your side at the level of your lower ribs. Slip your hand through the handle, palm facing up.

2 Roll onto your side so your whole body faces the bell. Grab the handle with your other hand, keeping your elbow against your lower ribs.

3 Roll onto your back again. Your elbow should be on the floor and bent 90 degrees, your forearm should be vertical and below your chest, and the bell should be resting against the back of your forearm. Your palm should face across your body, not toward your feet or head. The inside of your upper arm should touch your side. Don't let your forearm bend such that the bell comes closer to your face.

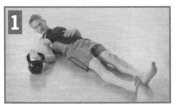
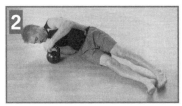
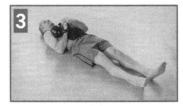

USING TWO BELLS:

1 Position a bell on either side of your body so that they're about a foot from you at the level of your lower ribs. Get one bell into position as noted above.

2 Keeping the first bell tight to your body, roll to the other side (the first bell must come with you). Slip your free hand into the second bell and bring your first hand as close as possible to the other hand.

3 Staying tight, roll onto your back again and bring the second bell into position with your forearm vertical, elbow on the floor, and bell on the outside of your forearm. Your palms are now facing each other, not pointing toward your feet or head. Don't let the elbows flare out. Your inner arms should be touching your sides.

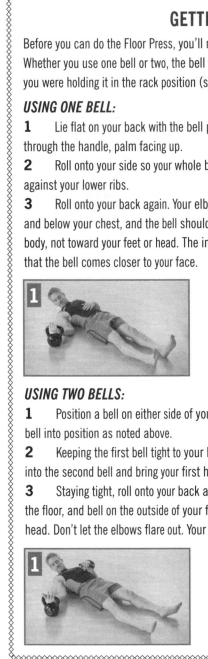
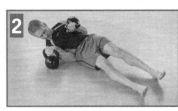
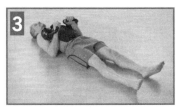

Rows

Kettlebell Rows are done a little differently than dumbbell rows. Most people use the shoulder too much when doing dumbbell rows by pulling the weight straight up. With the kettlebell, focus on total body strength and control and pull with the lats and upper back muscles. The obliques are also worked hard if you use the right weight and prevent rotation of the torso and shoulders.

ROW

STARTING POSITION: Place your left foot forward and your right foot back, with your feet about hip-width apart or slightly wider. The bell should be placed in line with the toes of your left foot and with the handle parallel to the foot; the bell should also be in the same line as your shoulder, not right next to your foot. Keep your back flat. Now place your left forearm across your left thigh, just above your knee. Grab the handle by the front corner of the bell with your right hand. Tip the bell so it rests on the back bottom edge of the bell.

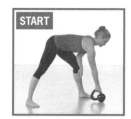

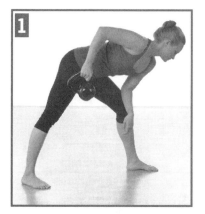

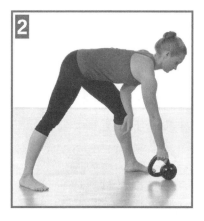

1 Focusing on using your back muscles and retracting your shoulder blade, squeeze everything tight and pull the bell to your hip. Don't let your shoulders or hips turn, or let your torso move up and down. Everything must stay locked in place in order to maximize the benefits from this lift.

2 Slowly return the bell to its starting position on the floor; it should lightly touch the floor. If the bell hits the floor hard, the bell is too heavy for you or you're being sloppy.

Things to consider:

• *How far apart you place your feet depends on your flexibility. Some people can get down fairly deep with the left thigh almost parallel to the floor. Others may need to keep their feet closer together, which alters the angle of the hips to feet. Regardless, keep your back flat and chest out.*

Slingshots

The *Slingshot*, or Around-the-Body Pass, is a nice ab exercise that also requires focus, coordination and kinesthetic awareness (i.e., knowing where your hands and feet are without being able to see them). It's great for active rest between more difficult exercises. Ideally, the only movement other than the arms comes from the ankles as you sway to counterbalance against the bell.

SLINGSHOT

STARTING POSITION: Stand with your feet together and hold the bell with both hands in front of you. The arms are hanging down, elbows straight.

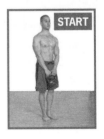

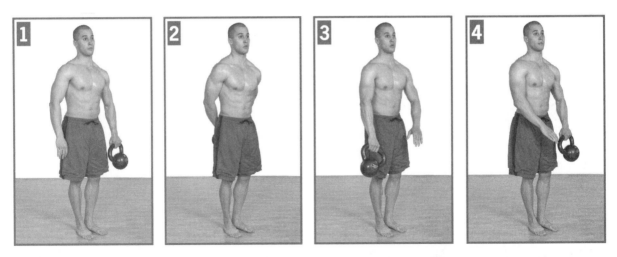

1–2 Release the bell from one hand and move both arms behind you, one to each side. As you do the Slingshot, your hands will always face the rear.

3 Without moving your torso, bending at your ribs or twisting, use your free hand to grab the handle by the open corner and release the other hand. Keep your abs, glutes and lower back locked together throughout the movement to prevent your torso from bending or turning.

4 Bring both arms back to the front and transfer the bell to the other hand.

Continue passing the bell around your body, then switch directions.

Figure 8s

The *Figure 8* involves threading the bell between your legs in—you guessed it—a figure-8 pattern. Since it's a fast-moving drill, it's easy to miss a transfer and drop the bell. If that happens, don't worry; just make sure you get your feet out of the way. Use a moderate-weight bell.

The *Figure 8 with a Tap* starts like the Figure 8 but adds a rotational hip pop to bring the bell up in front of the body. Most people get mixed up at first, so take your time and stay light. The hand switch occurs behind the knee, not in front of the chest, and the bell always passes from front to back through the legs.

FIGURE 8

STARTING POSITION: Stand with your feet about shoulder-width apart and hold the bell in your left hand so that the pinky part is in the corner of the bell with your palm facing back. Push your hips back like you're going to do a swing. Keep your chest up, back flat and abs tight throughout this exercise.

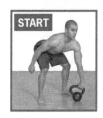
START

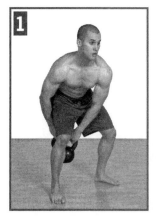
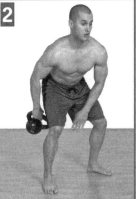
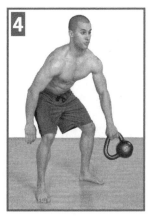

1–2 Thread the bell between your legs and transfer it to your right hand when the bell is behind your right knee. Both palms should face back at the time of transfer, and your thumbs should come together as the bell moves from one hand to the other.

3–4 Bring the bell around to the front and pass it back through your legs to the left and switch hands behind your left leg.

FIGURE 8 WITH A TAP

STARTING POSITION: Stand with your feet about shoulder-width apart and hold the bell in your right hand so that the pinky part is in the corner of the bell with your palm facing back. Push your hips back like you're going to do a swing. Keep your chest up, abs tight and back flat throughout this exercise. Your torso should naturally rotate toward the side the bell is moving.

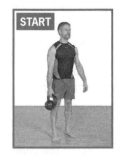

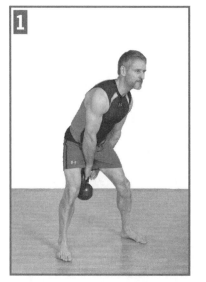

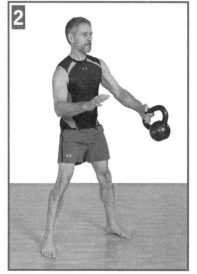

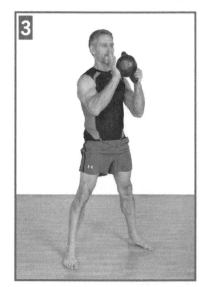

1 Pass the bell between your legs to your left hand when the bell is behind your left knee. The torso is rotated so the right shoulder is forward and the left back.

2–3 As the bell comes around your left knee, pop your hips and use your abs to stand up quickly, whipping the bell up. The power comes from the unwinding of the torso back to a fully erect, forward-facing body. Let your elbow bend and keep it close to your side, but don't use your arm to bring the bell up. When you're standing tall, your left palm should be facing you and your right hand (palm outward) should come up at the same time to stop the bell from crashing into your chest or shoulder.

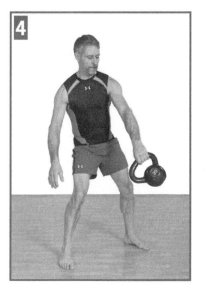

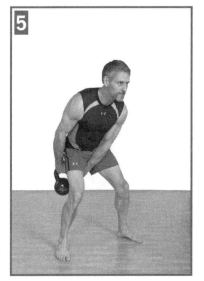

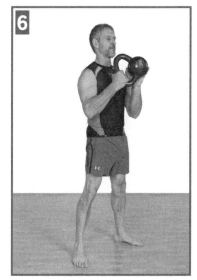

4 Push the bell out in front a little and rotate your left forearm so that the thumb points back to the right rear. Push your hips back and let the bell fall through your legs; your left shoulder is forward and your right is back. When it's behind your right knee, grab the bell with your right hand, letting the thumbs meet when the transfer occurs.

5-6 As the bell clears your right knee, whip it up using your abs and hips and stand up, unwinding your torso to come up standing tall, facing forward. Your right palm will be facing you about chest high and your left hand (palm facing out) will act as a block.

Push the bell away from your body, take your hips back and repeat.

Renegade Row

Renegade Rows are a fairly advanced movement in that you have to be able to support yourself on one arm. These can be dangerous if you lose focus; the bell will shift and fall and so will you. You'll need a pair of the same bells. This exercise marks the beginning of more advanced kettlebell lifts that require much more focus and attention to detail. You have to be patient and really practice them, staying on the lighter side until you've gained a decent level of control and understanding of each lift. Make sure you have a firm grasp of the beginner- and intermediate-level lifts before working with advanced movements. Some of these can be dangerous and a slight misalignment can cause a big injury.

ADVANCED

RENEGADE ROW

STARTING POSITION: Position the bells so that the handles are shoulder-width apart and parallel to your body. Place the hip of each hand (at the base of the little finger) on a handle and wrap your fingers around it; this grip will help keep your wrists straight. Now assume a good high plank/push-up position and lock out your hips.

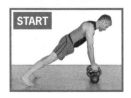

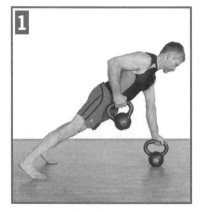

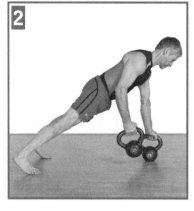

1 Keeping everything tight, especially your hamstrings, glutes, quads and abs, and locking out your supporting wrist, slowly pull one bell up to your hip. Note: any movement of the supporting arm or hand can cause the bell to tip over, making you fall. Avoid letting your hips come up and avoid rotating your hips or torso.

2 Slowly lower the bell back to starting position.

Shift your weight to the other arm and lock out everything before slowly pulling the other bell to your hip.

MODIFICATION: If you can't prevent your hips from coming up or your hips/torso from rotating, move your feet farther apart. If you still can't do it, use lighter bells or do it without bells. See page 115 for bodyweight rows.

Snatches

The snatch takes the kettlebell from the floor or between the legs to overhead in one fluid movement with no pressing, with the elbow locked and hand directly over the shoulder. There is more shoulder involvement as well as hand and forearm work in the snatch than the clean, but the majority of the work should be done with the legs—squat down and explode up. There are three variations: *Dead Snatch*, *Hang Snatch*, and *Swing Snatch*.

Usually done for exercise, the snatch is also a competition lift. The sport of kettlebell lifting (commonly referred to as "GS," short for "Girevoy Sport"; *girevik* is Russian for "weight lifter") focuses on snatches and double jerks in one event and the double clean and jerk (not discussed in this book) as a separate event. Competitors in the grueling snatch and double jerk competition (commonly referred to as the "biathlon") must snatch a bell for 10 minutes and cannot set it down during that time. They're only allowed to change hands once so their strength and endurance must be at a very high level. Male competitors must use a 32k (70lb) bell in order to achieve higher-level rankings in the sport.

The techniques used in GS are different from what is used by most practitioners for exercise and power development, but don't get hung up on one way being better than another. GS technique teaches you to develop power as well as sustain it for 10 minutes. "Hard style," as it has come to be known, is more focused on fast, explosive power in short bursts. The snatch portion of a workout is usually under five minutes and generally tries to get maximum reps in as short a time as possible. Many times, a hard-styler will tend toward doing sets and reps rather than timed intervals. Choose the style that aligns with your goals.

GETTING IN POSITION

There are two ways to get the bell overhead with the elbow locked out and the bell resting on the forearm. In the *first method*, keep your thumb pointed backward during the pulling phase and shove your hand through the handle at the top, the same thing you did for Dead Cleans (page 52); the bell will wrap around your wrist. The *second method*, which tends to be used more during "hard-style" snatches, involves punching your hand through the handle of the bell so it goes right over your fist, but there's no banging. Punching through changes the center of mass between the bell and your fist and lets the bell almost roll over your hand. However, your grip must be relaxed, just enough to hold onto the bell. If you squeeze too hard or don't punch through fast enough, the bell won't be able to rotate over your fist and will bang your forearm.

THE LOCKOUT

The top position of the snatch is referred to as the "lockout." The bell and arm are in the exact same place as in a press: The hand, turned slightly toward the body, is directly over the shoulder; the shoulder sits tight in the socket; and the bell rests diagonally across the palm, from the webbing between the thumb and index finger to the base of the little finger (the hip of the hand). You can keep your hand open or closed. Your biceps should be in line with your ear but there should be space between them. This is the exact same position as the press.

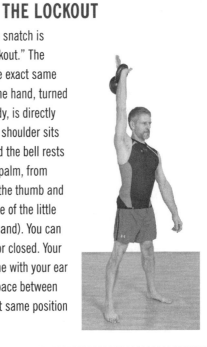

CARING FOR YOUR HANDS

Kettlebell practice can be tough on the hands. You'll get calluses, you'll get blisters or, worse, blisters under your calluses. Here are some tips to help you keep your hands in good shape.

- Use a file if your calluses aren't too tough, or use a "ped-egg" to keep your calluses smooth. If you trim or file them, it's best to do so in or just after taking a shower or bath. I remove calluses using a foot callus remover that has a curved razor blade in the handle by slicing them off. Be careful and don't go too deep. You just want to keep the calluses smooth and flat.

- Use a high-quality hand lotion or coconut oil on your hands. Coconut oil is better as it has antibacterial properties.

- If you do get a blister, don't pop it! It'll pop on its own. When it does, cut away the loose skin. As the rest of it loosens, trim it back as well. A blister will take five days or so to heal.

- If you do tear your hands, trim the loose skin off and use coconut oil to keep it from drying out and splitting. Tearing up your hands will keep you from training for several days.

- Don't use "Nu-skin" or similar products. It's basically super glue. Using it won't help your hands heal any faster.

- Some people ask about wearing weight lifting gloves to protect their hands, but I prefer my clients to not use any type of glove as it alters the grip and actually makes it harder to master the technique. However, if you have a job that requires delicate hands, then you may wear hand protection, but not weight lifting gloves—they're too thick. Get a pair of brown, cloth gardener's gloves and cut off most of the fingers, or take an old crew sock and cut holes for your fingers. These are thin enough to allow you to feel the bell but not thick enough to affect your grip much.

If you choose to use the rotation method like you did with the clean, start your snatches with your hand in the same position as in the Dead Clean. If you choose the punch-through method, hold the bell as you would with a 1-Hand Swing (page 43).

Snatches are a tough technique to master and thus require a lot of practice. Like the clean, focus on practicing the movement, not making a workout out of it. Stay with a moderate weight, usually one size up from what you normally press and work with it.

KEY POINTS FOR ALL SNATCHES

- The whole movement is one smooth, fluid, continuous action. There's no jerkiness and you shouldn't be getting banged in the forearm by the bell. Think of it as throwing the bell straight up as high as you can from the ground up and then punching through at the top as your elbow locks.

- Typically, people who use the punch-through method tend to keep their hand closed at the top, but it doesn't matter if you keep your hand open or closed in lockout. The bell should be on the back of your forearm at exactly the same time your elbow locks. If the bell is on your forearm before the elbow locks, you'll push the arm into lockout, involving your triceps.

- The lockout is caused by the hip drive and the arm whip, allowing the bell to wrap around the wrist or driving the hand through the handle. At no time should you feel like you're pressing the bell. If you feel it in your triceps, you're pressing it up, which means you're coming up slightly short in the movement.

- The bell *must* come off your palm and into your fingers as soon as you start to drop it, otherwise you'll tear up your hands. First the bell, then the hand, then the elbow, then the shoulder. Your knees bend and you start to squat as the bell starts to move below your elbow.

Like the Dead Clean, the Dead Snatch is fast and explosive—you *must* attack it. The distance you move the bell is more than double that of the clean, so don't expect to be able to Dead Snatch a really heavy (relative to your strength) bell initially.

STARTING POSITION: Place the bell on the floor between your feet as you would for Dead Cleans (page 52). Squat down and grab the handle with your left hand, using the Dead Clean grip or the 1-Hand Swing (page 43). Keep your torso upright and keep your elbow straight but "soft" at the start of each rep.

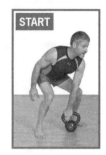

START

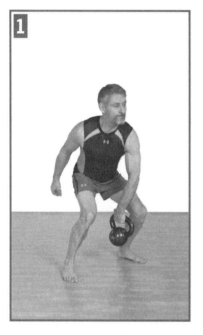

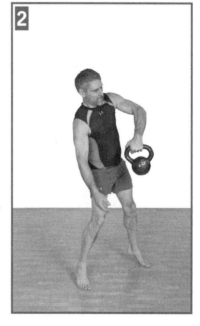

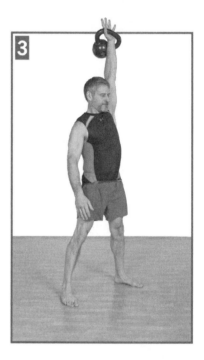

1–2 Keeping your arm as close to your body as possible without the bell hitting you, explode straight up and pull the bell off the floor. The bell's path is vertical. *If you're using the Dead Clean grip* (pictured), keep your thumb pointed toward you as the bell comes up. *If you're using the 1-Hand Swing grip*, keep your palm facing you as the bell comes up. As your hips extend, your shoulder rises, followed by your elbow, forearm, wrist, hand and bell. When your hips are fully extended, your shoulder should be at its highest point and your elbow should be higher than your shoulder.

3 As your forearm continues upward, your elbow straightens. When your forearm approaches vertical, flip your wrist so that your fingers point up. *If you're using the Dead Clean grip*, the bell should rotate around your wrist. *If you're using the 1-Hand Swing grip*, you'll have to be a little more aggressive with the flip or punch of the hand.

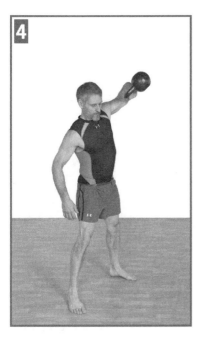

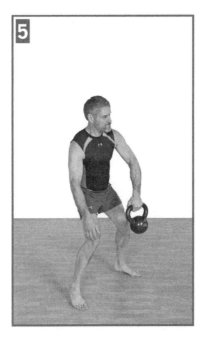

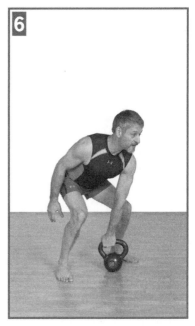

4 To return the bell to the floor, quickly bend your wrist so that your fingers point to the floor. As the bell comes off your hand, bend your elbow and let the bell fall into the crook of your fingers. *If you're using the Dead Clean grip,* wrap your thumb over your index finger and rotate your forearm so that your thumb points to your centerline; your thumb and forefinger take the brunt of the weight. *If you're using the 1-Hand Swing grip,* let the bell fall off the heel of your hand into the base of the fingers, keeping all fingers wrapped around the handle with your fist pointing back; all the fingers and thumb grip the bell.

5–6 As the bell falls, straighten out your arm and squat down, matching the speed of the bell with your legs so that your arm is straight when the bell lightly touches the floor. Keep your torso vertical. Use your legs to slow the bell, not your arm. The descent should be as smooth and fluid as the ascent of the bell.

The Hang Snatch is based on the same idea as the Hang Clean (page 54), except you take it overhead as you did in the Dead Snatch (page 86). The Hang Snatch is a shorter version of the Dead Snatch: You pull the bell a shorter distance and use a little more leg action, making it less difficult in terms of weight used (i.e., you can do the same weight you did in the Dead Snatch and it'll be easier or you can go up a size).

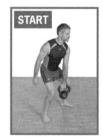

STARTING POSITION: Stand tall and hold the bell between your legs, using either the Dead Clean grip or 1-Hand Swing grip. Lower into a quarter squat.

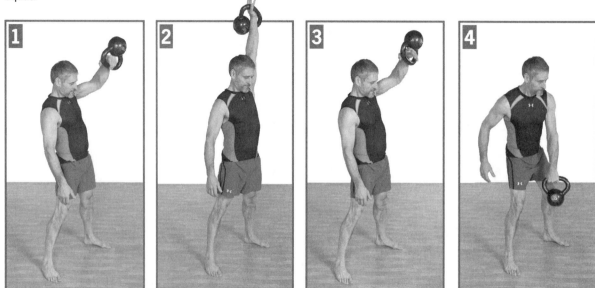

1 Pulling with your shoulder and using the upward momentum created by the knee dip and drive, rip the bell overhead. *If using the Dead Clean grip* (pictured), keep your forearm rotated so the thumb side of your hand points toward you. *If using the 1-Hand Swing grip*, keep your palm facing back. Your elbow will bend as your arm goes up; as the elbow goes above the shoulder, the forearm will go up and the elbow will straighten out.

2 Just before your elbow locks out, straighten your wrist so that your fingers point up. *If you're using the Dead Clean grip*, the bell should wrap around your fist. *If you're using the 1-Hand Swing grip*, drive your hand through the handle so that the bell rests again the back of your wrist.

3 To return the bell to hang position, tip your fingers and wrist down and get the bell off your palm and into your finger grip by popping your hand a little.

4 As the bell falls, match the speed of the bell by squatting so that your legs absorb the force of the falling weight. At the bottom, your arm should be fully straight and your knees should be bent in a quarter squat, ready to explode back up.

Pendulum or swing snatches (usually just called "snatches") can be performed "hard style" or "soft style" (see page 90). Don't get hung up on stylistic differences—use the method that best helps you meet your goals. If you use the same weight bell here as you did for the Dead Snatch (page 86) and Hang Snatch (page 88), you should find it takes much less effort to get the bell overhead.

STARTING POSITION: Swing the bell back between your legs just as you would with a 1-Hand Swing (page 43).

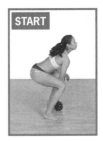
START

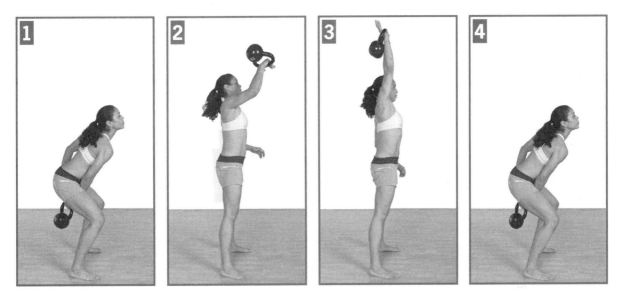

1–3 As the bell just passes forward through your legs, start to pull just like you did with the Hang Snatch—keep your arm in close, get your elbow up and let your forearm follow. Punch through the handle so the bell rests gently on the back of your forearm; your elbow should be locked, and the bell should be resting across your palm, from the webbing between your thumb and forefinger to the base of your little finger. Your shoulder should be packed down tight with your biceps by the ear but not touching.

4 Bring the bell back down like you did with the Hang Snatch, but redirect it between your legs (not down toward the floor) by pushing your hips back and bending your knees a little. You should now be in the same position as if you were doing a regular swing.

Use the momentum from the back swing and repeat steps 1–3 continuously. These movements should be very fast and powerful, but don't shortcut the movements. Make sure you get your arm all the way overhead.

exercise continued on next page

continued from previous page

Things to consider

- Keep your upper arm close to your body. The farther away from you the bell goes, the more impact to your wrist and forearm there will be at the top.

- Don't squeeze the handle too hard; squeeze it just enough to not drop it. Most hand issues are caused at the bottom of the movement, when the hands have to absorb the force of the bell falling. Learn to absorb with the legs and minimize hand involvement. Your hands have to become conditioned to the bell; every time you go up in weight, you increase the stress on your hands.

- If you're snatching a really heavy bell, use chalk to help your grip, especially if it feels like the bell is going to come out of your hand. The chalk is magnesium based for increased friction, as opposed to chalk used when playing pool. It's available at outdoor/climbing stores, online fitness stores and some sporting goods stores.

- Don't be in a hurry to snatch max weight or do long timed sets. There are various training protocols involved in both and you need to perfect your technique and let your hands get used to the work.

HARD STYLE VS. SOFT STYLE

There are several schools of thought on the best way to perform Pendulum Snatches. Some believe in what is called "hard style"—fast, explosive, powerful movements. Others espouse "soft style"—more relaxed and even paced, but still a powerful technique. In addition, within each "style" are some differences in how to best apply the methodologies. In my opinion, don't get hung up on stylistic differences—use the method that best helps you meet your goals.

Hard style will develop fast, explosive power over short work intervals, typically five minutes or less. The Pendulum Snatch done hard-style is as aggressive as a Dead Snatch—nothing but raw power. Soft style uses a longer but more relaxed stroke and stays a bit more relaxed in the effort, but make no mistake—soft style is still very powerful. Snatching a kettlebell for ten minutes with only one hand switch is very tough physically and mentally.

So why choose one over the other? If your goal is enduring strength, go with soft style. If you're after fast, hard, explosive power, use hard style. We cover only the hard-style snatch here.

You should've done the Dead Snatch (page 86) by now and have an idea of the raw power involved in ripping a kettlebell from the floor to overhead in a smooth, fluid movement. It's very powerful but still graceful. Adding a pendulum swing introduces sophistication to the movement—that is, you're now moving in two dimensions instead of one (behind you and overhead versus straight up). There are many variations in how much to swing it. We'll start with the method I think is best and easiest to figure out with minimal impact to the back of the forearm.

Start with a lighter bell and take your time learning the technique. Don't be in a rush to go heavy or fast too soon. This will also give your hands a chance to get conditioned to the work. This hand conditioning is important and, as you master the technique with one weight, you'll have to almost start over again when you increase it. Your hands have to get used to the heavier weight or you'll wind up tearing them up. (See page 84 for tips on how to take care of your hands.)

Alternating Cleans

The Alternating Clean requires a lot of coordination, timing and rhythm and is rather tough for some people. I don't recommend you try this until you have Dead and Hang Cleans down pat. There are actually two ways to do Alternating Cleans: 2-step and 1-step. The *2-Step Alternating Clean* is simpler and starts by holding both bells in hang position, cleaning one bell and returning it to hang, and then doing the same for the other bell. With *1-Step Alternating Cleans*, both bells move in opposite directions at the same time, with one being cleaned and the other being returned to the hang position. This is very demanding and hits the legs and abs especially hard; it also really increases your heart rate.

You'll need a pair of bells of the same size and weight.

STARTING POSITION: Stand tall and hold a bell in each hand between your legs.

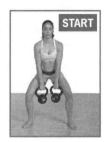

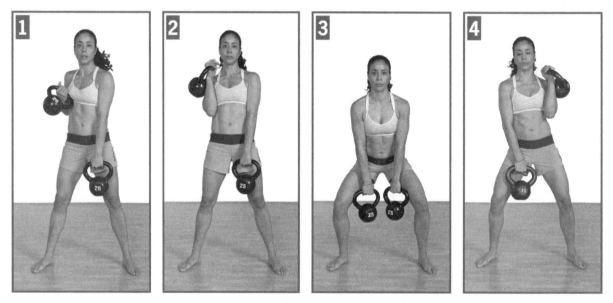

1–2 Bend your knees and explode up. Just as with the Hang Clean (page 54), your shoulder should naturally rise a little, followed by your arm and the bell. As your hips finish their upward movement, the bell should move straight up in front of your body. Keep your thumb turned toward you, quickly drop your elbow and drive your hand through the handle. You now have one bell in rack and one in hang position.

3–4 Dump the racked bell back to hang position, then clean the other bell. With the 2-Step Alternating Clean, there's a definite rest when you return the bell to hang.

1-STEP ALTERNATING CLEAN

You'll need a pair of bells of the same size and weight.

STARTING POSITION: Stand tall and hold a bell in each hand between your legs. Do a Hang Clean (page 54) with one bell so that one bell is racked and the other is in hang position.

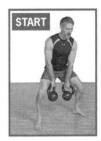

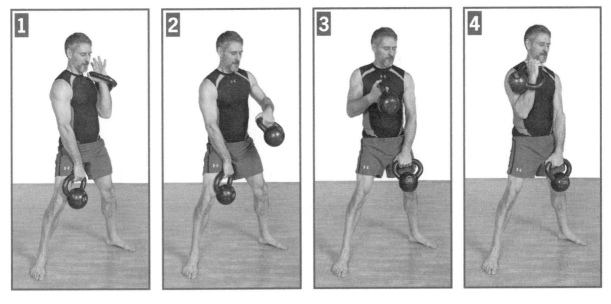

1–2 Dip your knees and hips and then explode up and clean the lower bell. As the lower bell begins to rise, the upper bell begins to fall.

3–4 As you finish the clean, bend your knees to absorb the fall of the upper bell, then drive up again and switch the bells. Focus on the bell going up; the one going down will take care of itself. Throughout this movement, your legs should continually pump up and down into a quarter squat and back to standing. There is no pause.

Turkish Getups

Reputedly Turkish Getups (TGU) originated in Turkey, but whether they did or not may never be known for sure. Regardless, the TGU is an awesome whole-body exercise. It works the shoulders, core and legs, and also improves athleticism, body control and awareness. The movement starts from the floor, flat on your back with a bell locked out (as in the Floor Press), to "getting up" and holding the bell locked out as though you just pressed it. It's truly a whole-body movement and works the core, shoulder, hamstrings, glutes and quads.

The TGU can be done several ways depending on your goals, the weight of the bell and whether you're using the movement to work on certain movement-quality issues like tight hip flexors. There are six primary positions to the TGU and most can be tweaked to suit your goals. Some of these pieces of the getup can be used as standalone exercises. For example, the first part of the TGU is a *Half Getup*. We also cover the *Getup Sit-Up* and the *Armbar*.

In addition to preparing you for the full TGU, the Half Getup is great for teaching you how to stabilize the shoulder of the arm that's up, strengthen the lower arm, drive your shoulder away from your ear and be fluid in your up and down movement. Do it slowly and with control on both sides, and you'll feel it in your shoulders, triceps and abs in the next day or so.

I usually teach the full TGU to my more advanced students and we start with no weight. When they show they can do the movement properly, I'll place a shoe on their fist. If they deviate from vertical, the shoe will fall. Then we go to a light bell and perfect the movement. Many times we'll work on just one part in each lesson, doing the first two steps for most of a session, then the next five steps the next time, and finally the last few steps from half kneeling to standing and back down. This creates and reinforces correct mechanics and gives students a sense of accomplishment and safety. They know and understand the movement and are comfortable with it before loading.

As the name implies, the Getup Sit-Up involves doing a sit-up with a kettlebell locked out. This works the core hard but also works your shoulder mobility, range of motion and static strength. The Armbar is an extended version of the initial roll from the back up to the forearm of the full TGU. Instead of coming up, you'll stay down and continue to roll, trying to get your chest on the floor. The Armbar is a great exercise for opening the chest, stretching the pecs and working on shoulder stability and mobility.

Gray Cook and Brett Jones created a two-disc DVD called *Kettlebells from the Ground Up* (available from DragonDoor.com) that covers all aspects of the TGU, so we'll just hit the main points here to make sure you do it safely. The main thing to remember is that, at all times, the arm holding the bell is locked and vertical—any deviation from vertical can cause you to drop the bell. If you have a partner, have them spot you.

TURKISH GETUP SPOTTER DIRECTIONS

It's important to have a spotter for the TGU when you're first learning it. The spotter needs to be positioned so that he can take the bell if necessary yet not impede the lifter's movement.

1 After the lifter does the initial floor press, stand to his side, close enough to keep your hands under the bell but not so close that the lifter is crowded.

2 Remain in place as the lifter goes into the hip bridge.

3 When the lifter begins to bring his front leg underneath, move so that you don't get in the way of his foot or leg.

4–5 As the lifter switches to the half kneeling position, move so that you're in line with the lifter's shoulder. Continue moving as the lifter stands.

Reverse the process when the lifter goes back down. You must remain aware of what the lifter is about to do and be careful not to trip over the lifter when repositioning.

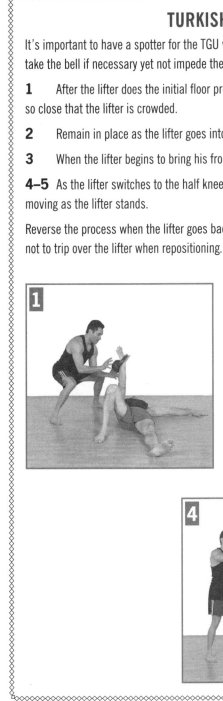
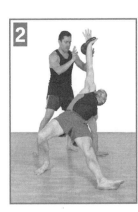
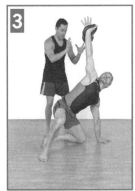

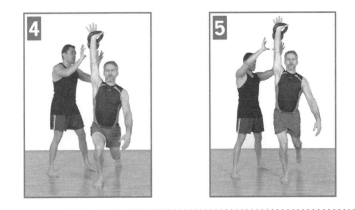

You should practice the Half Getup until you get the hang of it so you'll have a good base of support for the rest of the getup.

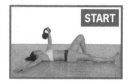

STARTING POSITION: Lie flat on your back and press a bell with your left arm, using the same technique as the Floor Press (page 75). Bend your left knee to about 45 degrees and make sure the foot is flat on the floor; your right leg remains straight along the floor. Your right arm is on the floor and out to the side approximately at shoulder level. Keep your left arm locked and vertical throughout the movement.

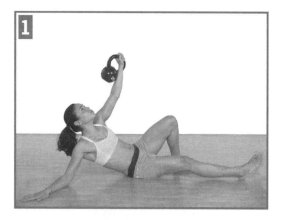

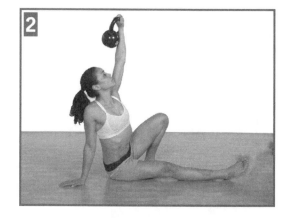

1-2 Driving with your left foot, roll from your upper right arm to your elbow and forearm so that you end up with your right palm flat on the floor supporting you and almost directly under your shoulder; your torso should be upright. Your left knee is still bent and pointing up, while your right leg is straight.

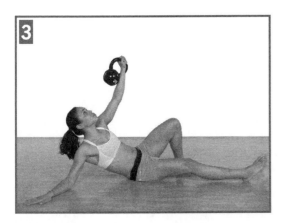

3 To return to your back, slowly slide your right arm out from under you toward the right rear (on the floor above your head to the right), letting your forearm, then your upper arm, roll to the floor.

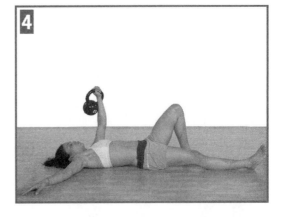

4 Once your right side comes into contact with the floor, roll onto your back and into starting position.

Start light! In fact, it's a good idea to first get used to the movement with either no weight or just a shoe balanced on your fist. If the shoe falls, you're not keeping your arm straight. Safety first!

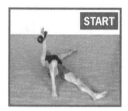

STARTING POSITION: Lie flat on your back and press a bell with your right arm, using the same technique as the Floor Press (page 75). Bend your right knee to about 45 degrees and place the foot flat on the floor; your left leg remains straight along the floor. Your left arm is on the floor and out to the side approximately at shoulder level. Keep your right arm locked and vertical throughout the movement.

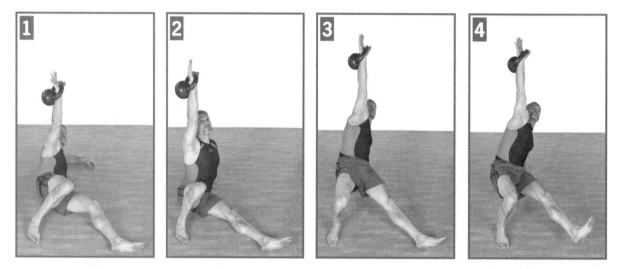

1–2 Driving with your right foot, roll from your upper left arm to your elbow and forearm so that you end up with your left palm flat on the floor supporting you and almost directly under your shoulder; your torso should be upright. Your right knee is still bent and pointing up, while your left leg is straight.

3–4 Driving your right heel into the floor, lift your butt off the floor as high as you can into a bridge position. Keep your hips facing the ceiling.

At the same time, drive your left shoulder into the floor by pushing the hand hard against the floor. Your left leg is still out in front but let it rotate from the hip so that the outside edge of the foot is on the floor.

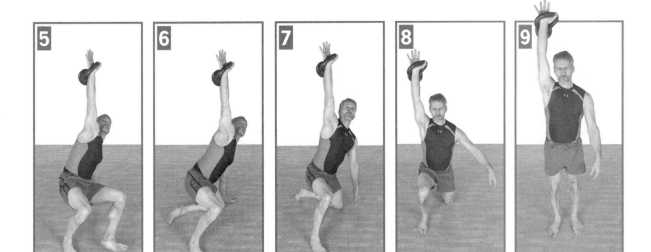

5–7 Bring your left leg under you, bending the knee and placing it just in front of your left hand. Your right shin is now close to vertical and your right foot is flat on the floor.

8 Swing your lower left leg out from under you and pivot on your knee so that your left foot is directly behind you; your torso should come up at the same time. You're now in a half kneeling position.

9 Flip onto the ball (rather than the top) of your left foot (this may happen naturally) and drive from the heel of the front foot and the ball of the back foot for a scissor effect, bringing you to a stand. As you stand, bring your left foot forward next to your right foot. You should now be the same as if you had just pressed the bell overhead.

exercise continued on next page

continued from previous page

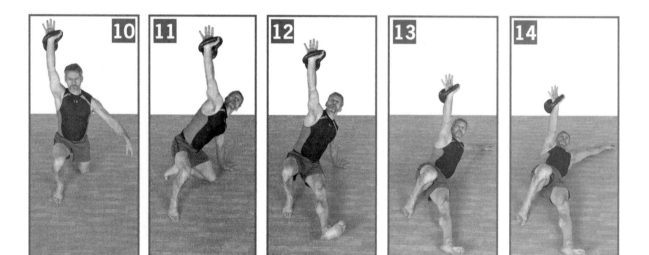

10 To return to the floor, step back with your left foot as in a back lunge and place your left knee gently on the floor.

11 Flip your left foot so that the top of the foot is on the floor. Rotating at the hip, swing your lower left leg under you so that your toes point to the right. At the same time, push your hips to the right and place your left hand on the floor by the left knee, driving your shoulder down away from your ear. Your right knee is bent and your shin is *almost* vertical with your right foot, which is flat on the floor.

12 Support yourself on your left hand and right foot. The right foot must stay flat on the floor; you may need to slide it forward about 2 to 3 inches to keep the heel down. Lift your hips and shoot your left leg out from under you, extending your knee and letting the outside of the foot rest on the floor.

13–14 Slowly slide your left arm out from under you toward the left rear. Let your forearm then your upper arm roll to the floor.

Your left side then comes into contact with the floor. Roll onto your back and into starting position.

From here, you have three options: 1) Bring the bell down to the floor, drag it to the other side and do a rep on the left; 2) leave your right arm extended and do another rep on the right; 3) or re-press the bell on the right and repeat the getup. Option 1 is usually used when going heavy, option 2 for when you're lifting light, option 3 for moderate weight (re-pressing the bell gives the shoulder a little rest but works the chest and triceps more).

Don't go too heavy on these or you could drop the bell.

STARTING POSITION: Take a heavy bell and stick your right foot through the handle so that your heel is on the ground. This gives you something to brace against during the rest of the movement. (You can also use a sandbag or even a heavy bag of dog food to anchor your foot.) Lie flat on your back and press a bell with your right arm, using the same technique as the Floor Press (page 75). Keep your legs straight and your elbow locked throughout the entire movement.

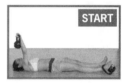

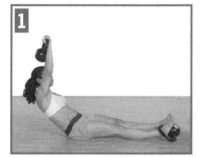

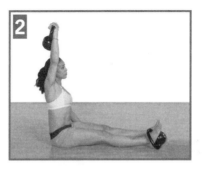

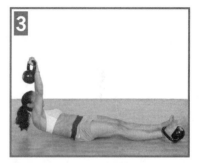

1–2 Sit up. As you do so, your arm will move slightly toward your toes; be sure to bring it back to vertical once you finish sitting up. Your body moves under your arm. Make sure you're sitting fully upright at the end of the sit-up; keep your shoulder packed in its socket. Keep your abs tight and stick out your chest.

3 Slowly lower yourself to the floor, trying to curl through each vertebra.

Use the same technique to switch sides as you did in the Floor Press. There is no need to switch the anchoring bell.

Remember to stay light (even to the point of using a shoe or a can of soup) and go slow. Only do one or two reps at a time until you have good control and body awareness. Practice the movement and ease into it; you have no margin for error here. If you rush the movement or go too heavy, you may injure yourself. *Keep one eye on the bell at all times so you'll know if your arm is off vertical.* Look out of the corner of your eye and keep your neck straight.

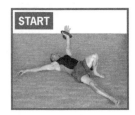

STARTING POSITION: Lie flat on your back and press a bell with your left arm, using the same technique as the Floor Press (page 75). Bend your left knee to about 45 degrees and place the foot flat on the floor; your right leg remains straight along the floor. Your right arm is on the floor and out to the side approximately at shoulder level. Keep your left arm locked and vertical throughout the movement.

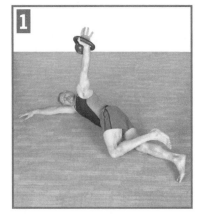

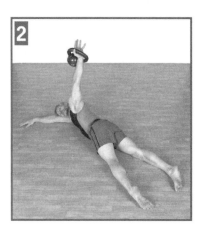

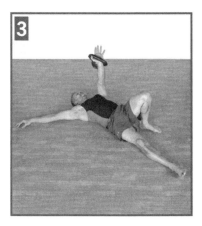

1 Push with your left leg and roll your body to the right. As you roll, bring your right arm above your head so that you can rest your head on the inside of your upper arm.

2 Bring your left leg over your right and straighten it out to get your chest on the floor, or as close as possible. Hold the position for 2 or 3 seconds, working the stretch and stabilizing the shoulder.

3 Slowly bring your left leg back to starting position to roll onto your back.

Windmills

The Windmill strengthens the shoulder while working mobilization, stretches the hamstrings and glutes, teaches whole body awareness and control, and hits the abs (especially the obliques) hard. There are three versions of the Windmill: *Low*, *Overhead* (sometimes referred to as the High Windmill) and *Double*. In the Double Windmill, you combine the Low and High Windmills into one exercise.

The Overhead Windmill is an awesome exercise if done correctly but can be dangerous if you get out of alignment. You may want to have someone compare your form to the photos in this book, paying particular attention to keeping a straight spine and not reaching out in front of you (your shoulders and hips stay almost parallel). The body mechanics of the Overhead Windmill are the same as the Low Windmill, except the muscles involved are different. The Low Windmill is a strong lower ab activator. The Overhead Windmill also uses those muscles but is more about shoulder mobility and stability. You'll also work the hamstrings and glutes harder because you move deeper into the stretch. You can work on Double Windmills once you've mastered the Low and Overhead Windmills since this Windmill combines the other two into one exercise.

Regardless of the version you do, you should move in a slow, controlled manner. Don't rush things and don't worry about using heavy bells. So you don't get hurt, keep on the lighter side until you've mastered the movements. Remember, safety first!

STARTING POSITION: Stand with your feet about shoulder-width apart. Place a bell on the floor next to the instep of your left foot. Rotate your left hip so that the foot and knee point about 45 degrees to the left. Your right foot can either point straight ahead or also to the left. Hold your right arm straight up so that your hand is over your shoulder and your elbow is locked; try to keep it vertical throughout the movement.

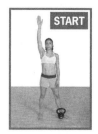

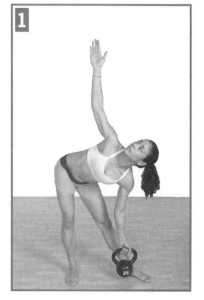

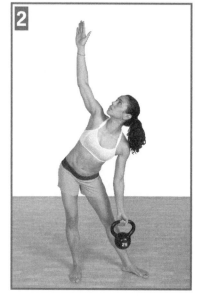

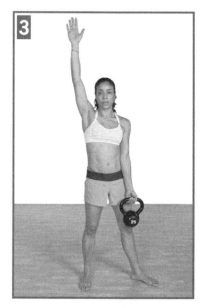

1 Keeping your chest lifted and your spine straight, push your hips hard to the right and fold through the hips. Make sure your hip goes to the side, not to the rear, to prevent upper body rotation. Let your left arm slide down the inside of your leg until you can grasp the bell's handle in your left hand. Although your right arm should remain vertical the whole

time, let it rotate a little as you go down, moving your body around your shoulder joint. Your knees should be straight or close to it; try to keep your right knee straight even if you have to bend your left knee a little. Keep your weight centered over your right leg.

2–3 Holding onto the bell with your left hand, stand up by reversing the hip movement. You should feel this in your obliques, hamstrings and glutes.

Repeat by pushing your hips back to the right, lowering the bell to the floor by the arch of your foot and standing back up.

OVERHEAD WINDMILL

Keep your upper arm as close to perfectly vertical as possible or else you'll lose control and drop the bell. Also, don't try to exceed your range of motion. Initially, you may want to try this with no weight or a very light one.

STARTING POSITION: Stand with your feet about shoulder-width apart and get the bell overhead by doing a clean and press or a snatch with your right arm. Position your feet so that they're the same as when you squat, then turn your left foot toward the left about 45 degrees and your right foot slightly to the left as well.

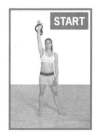
START

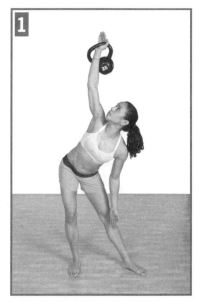

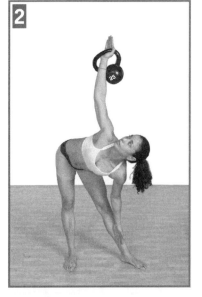

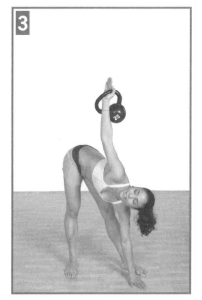

1–2 Keeping an eye on the bell and your shoulder in its socket at all times, push your hips hard to the right and let your left arm slide down the inside of your left leg, going as deeply as you can. Keep your chest lifted, your spine straight, your core tight and your knees, especially the right one, straight.

As you fold down, let your arm rotate in its shoulder socket so that your hand goes from facing forward to facing almost to the rear. Your right shoulder rotates clockwise while your left rotates counterclockwise.

3 Touch the floor with your left hand if possible, but don't lose your form. To come up, lift

your torso by squeezing your glutes, abs and hamstrings and return to standing position. Your shoulder unwinds so that your palm is facing forward again.

When you're done, bring the bell back to rack then place it on the ground, just as though you were finishing a Dead Clean.

You'll need two bells (I recommend a light bell for overhead and a slightly heavier one for the floor until you're very comfortable with this exercise). If you feel confident in your shoulders, you can use the same weight for both arms, but I wouldn't go heavy on top and light on the bottom until you become very proficient with this variation.

STARTING POSITION: Stand with your feet about shoulder-width apart. Place the bottom bell by the instep of your left foot and rotate your left leg about 45 degrees to the left. Get the other bell overhead by cleaning and pressing or snatching it.

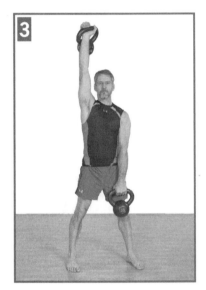

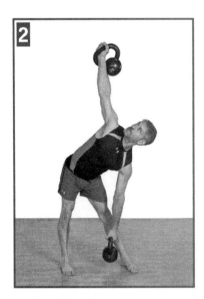

1 Keeping your spine and both knees straight, push your hips hard to the right and fold through your hips. Slide your left arm down the inside of your left leg. Allow your right shoulder to rotate in its joint so that your palm faces to the outside. Keep your weight on your right leg.

2–3 Once you can touch the lower bell, grab it with your left hand and drive off your right leg, using your abs, glutes and hamstrings, to move your torso back into position. Stand up tall with your right arm locked out and packed in the shoulder. Your left arm will be hanging between your legs, elbow straight and shoulder in its socket.

Repeat by pushing your hips back to the right, lowering the bell to the floor while keeping your right arm vertical; your right hand will face the rear. When you're finished, lower the upper bell to rack, then between your legs, then set both bells down.

Jerks

The jerk is an overhead movement in which you bring the bell from the rack to lockout and back to rack by using the legs to drive the bell up. You then drop under/away from the bell as it goes up, and then finally stand up. The actual lockout must occur when the elbow is straight, just as with the snatch; however, with the jerk the knees bend when the elbow locks. To finish the lift, you must stand and lock the knees after the arm is locked out.

This rather tricky movement is all about the legs. It develops strong, explosive lower body power, which translates well into activities that require a lot of jumping, sprinting and kicking. The idea behind the jerk is to use as much leg power and as little arm power as possible. You can jerk a lot more weight than you can press. You may be able to push press more than you can jerk, though, mostly because the jerk requires greater flexibility and coordination than the push press. The push press is a less sophisticated movement. When doing the clean and jerk, or long cycle (LCCJ), the clean helps you get a brief rest and also lets you reset your position. However, the extra movement requires more energy.

There are a lot of tweaks and tips that competitors use to maximize their efficiency when doing jerks, most of which are beyond the scope of this book. We'll give you the basic steps to performing the jerks and focus on getting the coordination down. From there, you can explore further by going online for more information.

For simplicity, we're only going to discuss the 1-Arm Jerk. The clean and jerk simply adds a clean to each rep. The technique for double jerks and double clean and jerks are the same as their single counterparts. Double jerks are very tough, especially when practicing for timed sets. Two bells resting in rack against the chest makes it very tough to breathe, even more so if you're already fatigued. If you study BJJ or other grappling arts including wrestling, you know how hard it is to breathe when someone is lying across your chest. Practicing holding two bells in rack while fatigued will help you in those other sports.

When doing double LCCJ you may find you have to move your feet around a lot. Typically you have to have a wider stance when cleaning two bells than one bell, but the wide stance will negatively impact the effectiveness of your leg drive; therefore, you have to continually adjust your stance. As the bells come up from between your legs, bring your feet under your hips. Of course, when you re-clean the bells, you have to move the feet apart again. This constant stance adjustment further adds to the fatigue of doing double LCCJ.

Keep in mind that this is an extremely fast, powerful movement. So while we go step by step, you're really moving with fluidity, grace and power.

STARTING POSITION: Stand with your feet about hip-width apart. Clean the bell to rack position, keeping your elbow in tight to your ribs. Stand tall and keep your knees straight, but don't squeeze your quads hard.

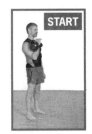

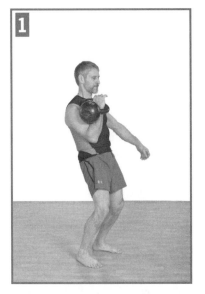

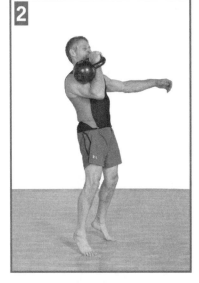

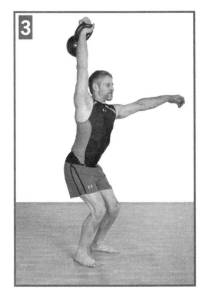

1 Push your hips forward and down and let your knees bend as deeply as possible while keeping your feet flat on the floor. Don't squat—your hips go forward during this phase (called the "first dip").

2 Driving from your feet, explode up, extending your hips and coming up on the balls of your feet. Your arm should float up from the force of the leg drive. Don't push with your arm.

3 As the bell rises, and just before your hips finish extending, drop quickly into a partial squat (called the "second dip") and lock your elbow. The idea is to get under the bell to lock your elbow, not to press it to lockout.

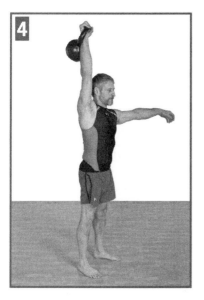

4 Stand up and lock your knees to complete the rep.

5 To return to rack, let your elbow bend and the bell fall straight down. At the same time, come up on the balls of your feet and meet the falling bell with the front of your deltoid.

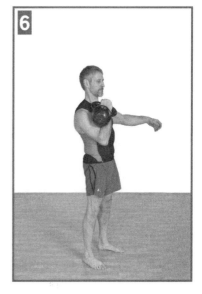

6 Let the bell slide from your deltoid to rack position and at the same time return to a flat-foot position. You should now be back where you started the jerk.

To do another jerk, explode up; to do LCCJ, re-clean the bell.

Things to consider:

• The farther apart your feet are, the less drive you get from your legs.

• The more powerful the initial dip and drive, the less you'll need to squat. If your initial drive isn't strong enough, you'll have to squat more in the second dip.

• Returning the bell to rack quickly and efficiently after a rep is almost as important as being efficient in the jerk itself. The faster you can hit lockout, get the rep count and return to rack the better. Minimize the time the bell is overhead and you can do more work.

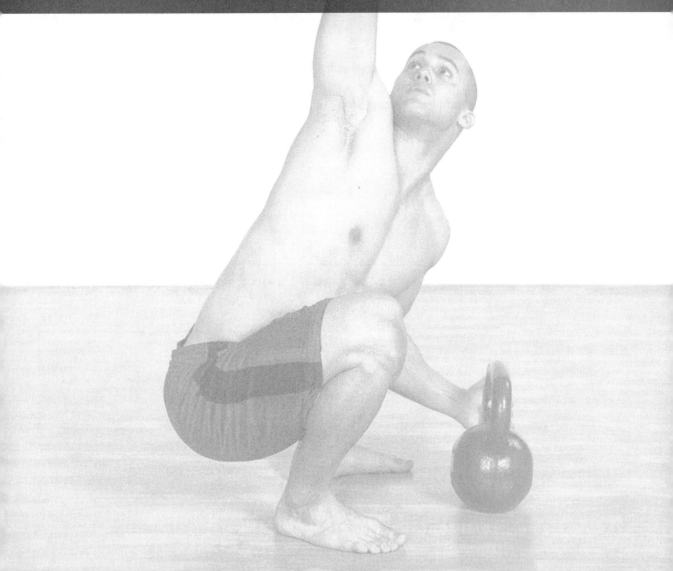

PART 4

APPENDIX

Warm-Ups

Warming up for kettlebell practice should be just like warming up for anything else. Go slow and easy and work your way into more intense activity as your muscles get warm and your blood flows. What you don't want to do are static stretches where you hold a position, trying to get the muscle to relax. This type of stretch is great after a tough workout but is actually detrimental to performance when done prior to a workout. You want the muscles to become warm and active, not cooled off and relaxed.

Here are some good bodyweight exercises that, when done slowly and deliberately, make for a great whole-body warm-up.

PUSH-UP

STARTING POSITION: Place your hands on the floor so that they're under your shoulders. Step your feet straight back and lock out your hips. This is the plank position. You should have a straight line from the back of your head to your feet.

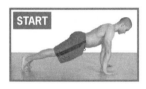

1 Keeping your elbows by your sides, slowly lower down until your triceps and lats touch. Don't let your belly sag.

2 Push the floor away to return to top position.

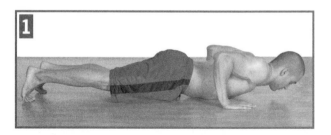

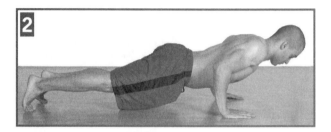

HIGH PLANK: STATIC HOLD

1 Assume the top push-up position. Hold this position for as long as you can.

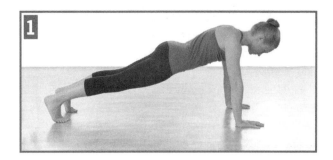

MIDDLE PLANK: STATIC HOLD

1 From the top push-up position, lower yourself halfway down and hold for as long as you can. Keep your elbows by your sides and your whole body tight.

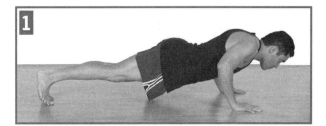

LOW PLANK: STATIC HOLD

1 From the top push-up position, lower yourself until you're at the bottom of a push-up. Hold for as long as you can, keeping your whole body tight.

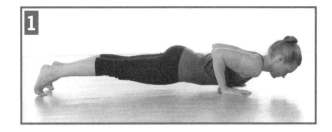

PARTIAL LOWER FROM HIGH PLANK

1–2 From the high plank, slowly lower yourself, leading with your chest, not your hips. Keep your elbows pointing toward the rear; don't let them flare out to the sides. Again, keep everything tight. When you can't go any lower without compromising your form, hold that position as long as you can then slowly raise back up.

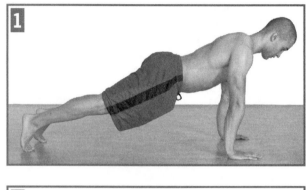

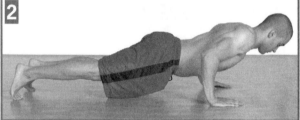

PARTIAL RAISE FROM LOW PLANK

1–2 From the low plank position, squeeze as hard as you can and try to lift yourself off the floor. Do not lift your chest independently from the rest of your body. Keep everything rigid and move your entire body as a unit. Go as high as you can, hold the position for as long as possible and lower yourself slowly, maintaining proper form the entire time.

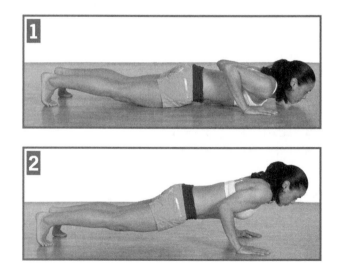

MOUNTAIN CLIMBER

STARTING POSITION: Assume a high plank with one knee tucked under you. You'll be supporting your weight with your upper body throughout the movement. Keep your elbows locked and hands shoulder-width apart.

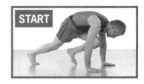

1–2 Switch feet by quickly driving the tucked knee back and pulling the other knee under you. Your feet should not slide along the floor. The only time your feet touch the floor is the split second when one knee is up under you and the other leg is fully extended. As soon as you hit that position, move right through it and keep going.

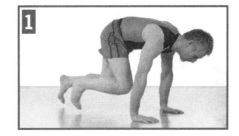

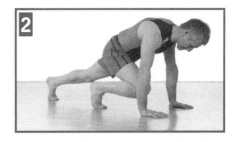

RENEGADE ROW (BODYWEIGHT)

STARTING POSITION: Assume a high plank.

1 Pull one hand back to your hip, utilizing your lats to retract your shoulder blade. Make sure you keep your hips and abs tight—there should be no rotation in the hips or waist.

Lower your hand and repeat on the other side.

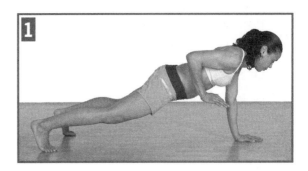

Burpees dynamically combine a squat, a push-up or plank, a double-knee tuck and potentially a jump squat.

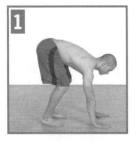 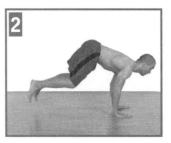 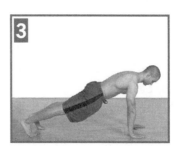 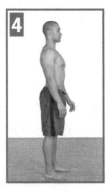

1 Squat and put your hands on the floor.

2–3 Kick both feet back so you're in a solid push-up/high plank position. Try to keep your hips low.

4 Bring both knees back under you and shift from the balls of your feet to a flat foot position and stand. Upon standing, squat back down and repeat.

BURPEE LEVEL 2

For level 2, instead of standing at the end, jump up and reach for the sky. Land softly by absorbing into your legs and go right back to the floor. Your feet should make little to no noise; don't "stick" the landing like they do in gymnastics.

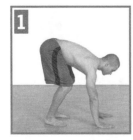 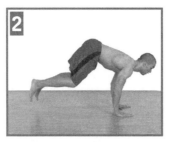 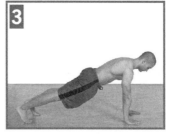 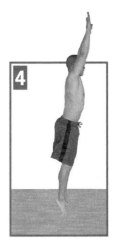

BURPEE LEVEL 3

For the full burpee, drop into a push-up instead of just putting your hands on the floor. Then, after you come to a plank position, do a push-up.

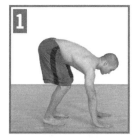

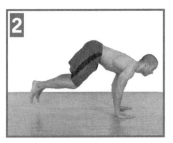

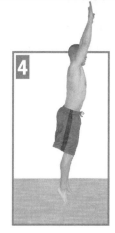

BOOTSTRAPPER

This is a bodyweight movement but you'll need a heavy bell to hold onto. The bootstrapper opens the hips, helps loosen up the lower back, and works on ankle mobility. If you're very flexible, you may be able to get into and hold the bottom position without holding the bell. If so, hold your toes.

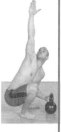

STARTING POSITION: Stand with your feet shoulder-width apart and place a bell out in front of them. Squat deeply, keeping an upright torso and your knees lined up with your toes. Hold onto the bell and sit back and down on your heels. Use your elbows to pry your knees apart. Find space in your hips.

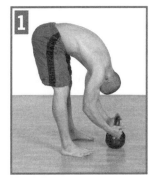

1 Still holding the bell, lift your hips up and let your head release to the floor. You're now stretching your hamstrings. Hold for a second and then pull yourself back down.

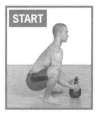

ADVANCED VARIATION: You must be able to keep your upper body vertical at the bottom of the bootstrapper to do this variation. From the start position, let go of the bell with one hand and open up your chest and shoulder by sweeping the arm up and out. As your arm goes up, rotate your neck so that you're following the arm with your head. Lower the arm to the bell, repeat with the other arm, then move to step 1 above. Repeat for 30 to 50 seconds.

This warms up the hip flexors, glutes and hamstrings. By adding an upper body rotation, you can continue to open the chest and back along with the lower body.

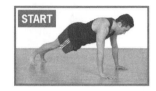

STARTING POSITION: Assume a push-up position, with your hands slightly wider than your shoulders, your elbows pointing back, your hands in line with your mid-chest (nipple line), and your feet hip-width apart. Keep your hips down and locked out so you have a straight line from the back of your head to the back of your feet.

1 Without lifting your hips, bend your right knee and bring your right leg close to and on the outside of your right hand. Hold the position for one to two seconds, feeling the stretch in the right hamstrings, right glutes and left hip flexor.

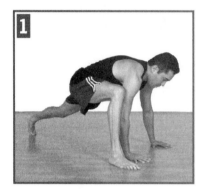

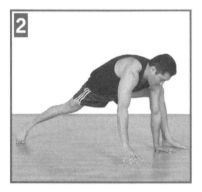

2 Return the leg to starting position and repeat with the other leg. Take your time; it's a hip opener, not an exercise.

ADVANCED TWIST VARIATION: Once your foot is next to your hand, rotate your torso and raise the arm that is next to the foot up to at least vertical. Keep your elbow straight throughout the rotation. The movement should occur in your mid-back, not in your lumbar spine.

SUPER-ADVANCED TWIST VARIATION: An even more advanced version is to rotate to the side opposite the foot (e.g., if your left foot is forward, rotate to the right) and raise the arm in an arc to vertical.

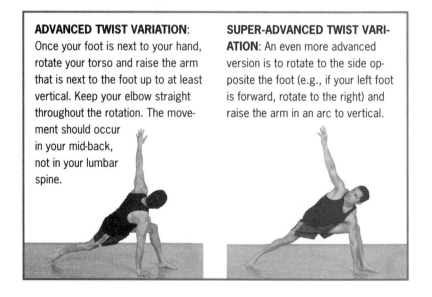

JUMPING JACKS

Jumping jacks are a great way to get your core temperature up, loosen the shoulders and hips, and work on staying soft and light-footed.

STARTING POSITION: Stand with your feet shoulder-width apart and arms by your sides.

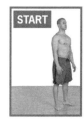

1 Jump your legs wider than shoulder-width apart while lifting your arms out to the sides and then overhead.

2 Quickly return your arms to your sides as you jump your feet back together.

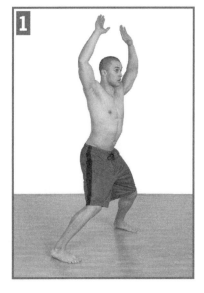

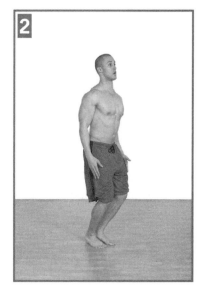

SCISSOR VARIATION 1: Move your legs out to the side while scissoring your arms across your body, alternating top hands.

SCISSOR VARIATION 2: Move your legs front to back while scissoring your arms across your body, alternating top hands.

SWING VARIATION: Move your legs front to back and raise one arm up overhead from the front while moving the other arm down to your rear.

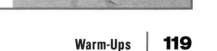

STARTING POSITION: Stand with your feet wider than shoulder-width apart, pointing your feet straight ahead as much as possible.

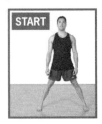

1 Keeping both feet flat on the floor, shift your weight to your right leg and keep your left leg straight. Sink your right hip to the rear and keep your chest up—don't bend over. Make sure your knees and toes remain in alignment. Don't let your shoulder lean past your weighted leg, and don't turn your hips or foot to the side.

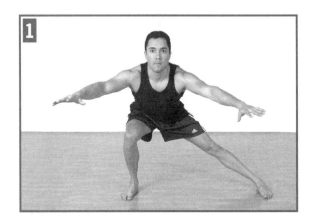

2 Keeping both feet flat on the floor, raise yourself back up and shift to the other side.

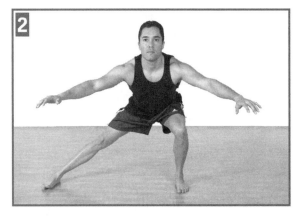

ADVANCED VARIATION: Shift side to side without coming up in between. This is more of a stretch for the inner thighs as opposed to a lunge.

SIDE-TO-SIDE STEPPING LUNGE

This is similar to the Side-to-Side Stretch Lunge (page 120) except for the middle movement. You can go slowly or you can go faster to work on dynamically loading and unloading the hips and weighted leg. The quick foot switch is an excellent way to improve your footwork for tennis, martial arts or any other sport that requires quick lateral direction changes.

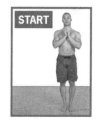

STARTING POSITION: Stand with your feet together, pointing your feet straight ahead as much as possible.

1 Keeping both feet flat on the floor and toes pointing forward as much as possible, step your right foot out to the right about 1.5 times wider than shoulder width. Sink your hips back and down. Make sure your right knee stays aligned with your right toes.

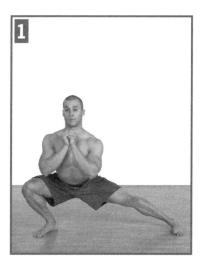

2 Drive off your right foot and return to standing.

3 Keeping both feet flat on the floor and toes pointing forward as much as possible, step out with your left foot to the left about 1.5 times shoulder width. Your left knee should be aligned with your left toes.

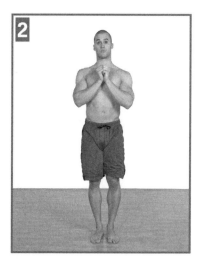

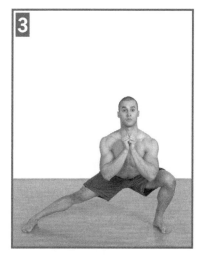

Whether you alternate legs or do one side repeatedly then the other, forward lunges mobilize the hip flexors and activate the gluteus maximus. It also hits the top of the thigh. Some trainers teach the forward lunge with the feet stepping out like you're on a tightrope. That's OK if you're very advanced and have excellent core control, but I prefer keeping the feet lined up with the hips. Hip-width lunges still require a lot of stabilization but there's less of a balance requirement.

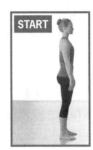

STARTING POSITION: Stand tall with your feet directly under your hips.

1 Leading with the heel, not the toe or ball of the foot, step your right foot forward, close to your normal walking stride. The heel of your front foot is firmly on the floor; your weight should not be on the ball of your foot. Keep the heel of your back foot up.

2 Now sink your hips straight down so that your front knee bends 90 degrees and your back knee almost touches the floor. There should also be a 90-degree bend in your front hip and your back hip; your back knee is bent almost 90 degrees. Keep your torso vertical with a tall spine. Your front shin should be vertical; don't allow it to shift forward.

3 To come up, drive straight up by simultaneously pushing into your front heel and the ball of your back foot. Once you're up, step your right foot back until both feet are under your hips.

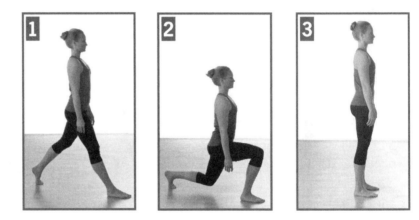

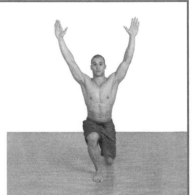

PRISONER'S VARIATION: To also open the mid-back, place your hands behind your head and interlock your fingers.

Y VARIATION: Try the lunge while holding your arms up, hands wider than shoulder width and shoulders in their sockets. This variation opens your mid-back, low back and shoulders, and improves ankle flexibility.

A static lunge is a forward lunge without the step, a regression in complexity of movement but tougher in terms of work done.

STARTING POSITION: Stand tall with your feet directly under your hips.

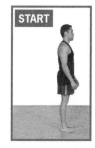

1 Leading with the heel, not the toe or ball of the foot, step your right foot forward, close to your normal walking stride. The heel of your front foot is firmly on the floor; your weight should not be on the ball of your foot. Keep the heel of your back foot up.

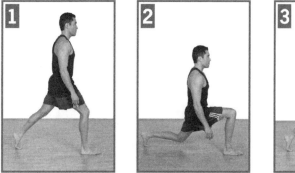
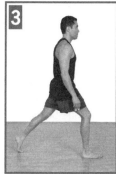

2 Now sink your hips straight down so that your front knee bends 90 degrees and your back knee almost touches the floor. There should also be a 90-degree bend in your front hip and your back hip; your back knee is bent almost 90 degrees. Keep your torso vertical with a tall spine. Your front shin should be vertical; don't allow it to shift forward.

3 To come up, drive straight up by simultaneously pushing into your front heel and the ball of your back foot.

Perform all reps on one side before switching legs.

PRISONER'S VARIATION: To also open the mid-back, place your hands behind your head and interlock your fingers.

Y VARIATION: Try the lunge while holding your arms up, hands wider than shoulder width and shoulders in their sockets. This variation opens your mid-back, low back and shoulders, and improves ankle flexibility.

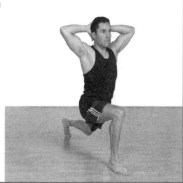

Bodyweight squats are done with the torso and shins as vertical as possible, with the movement starting by pulling the hips down and back.

STARTING POSITION: Stand with your feet about shoulder-width apart, feet pointing as straight ahead as possible (or up to 30 degrees out). Keep your weight on the mid to back part of your feet; you can lift your toes to make sure your weight is distributed properly. Pick a spot on the wall and focus on it. You can hold your arms out in front of you for balance.

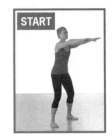

1 Contract your abs and use them and your hip flexors to pull your torso down, moving your hips down and back. Your hips move before your knees bend. Go as deeply as you can but don't tip over. Don't bend to get your head closer to the floor. Keep your shins as close to vertical as possible; don't push the knees forward.

2 To stand up, drive through your heels, lift your torso up as your hips rise and straighten your knees.

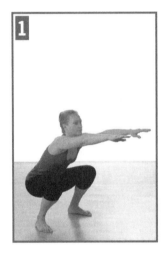

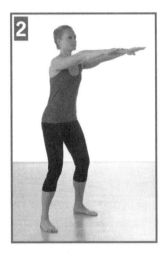

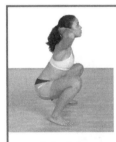

PRISONER'S VARIATION: You can also work on your mid- and upper-back mobility by first interlacing your fingers behind your head.

Y VARIATION: Before squatting, hold your arms up in a "Y," keeping your shoulders in their sockets. When you squat, try to keep your hands in line or slightly behind your ears while your elbows remain locked. This can also be done by holding a piece of PVC, a light resistance band or even a broomstick.

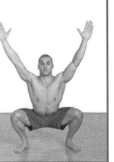

1-LEG STIFF-LEG REACH

This movement improves ankle stability, balance, core activation, glute activation and awareness of body position in space. If you do yoga, you might recognize this as Warrior 3.

STARTING POSITION: Stand with your feet under your hips and your arms by your sides.

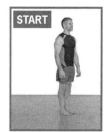

1 Slightly bend one knee, then slowly fold through your hips, raising your other leg behind you while at the same time raising your arms up in front of you, palms facing each other. Your goal is to be totally parallel to the floor from fingers to toes, including your hips.

2 Slowly lower your arms and leg and return to standing.

Switch sides or repeat on the same side for reps or time interval.

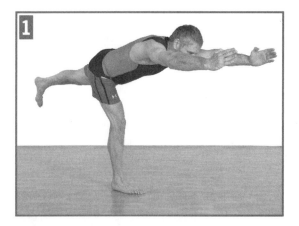

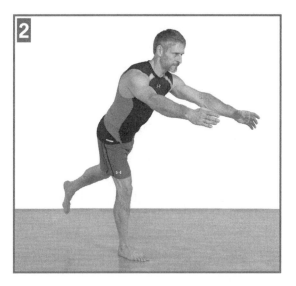

The Halo recruits the upper back and shoulders as well as the upper abs. It opens the shoulders and works on improving their mobility. This can be used as a warm-up or cool-down, although I occasionally use it during a workout. Use a light to moderate bell.

STARTING POSITION: Stand tall and hold the bell upside down in front of your sternum by the handle. The handle is parallel to your chest and your elbows are bent 90 degrees.

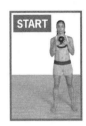

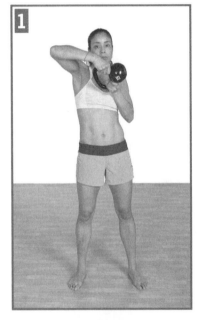

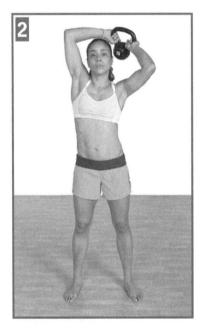

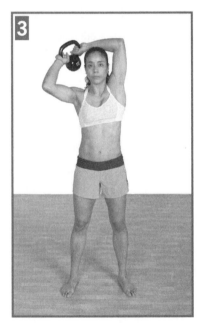

1–2 Maintaining the 90-degree bend in both elbows, rotate your arms at the shoulders so that your right arm goes up; pull the bell toward your left shoulder. As the bell approaches your left shoulder, your right forearm is parallel to the floor and will approach the top of your head.

3 Keep rotating through the shoulders, bringing your right forearm over your head so it just clears, brushing your hair. At the same time, the bell moves behind your head. Don't bend or twist your neck to get your head out of the way; stay tall. As your right arm passes your head, your left will come around behind so you

wind up with the bell behind your head, handle up and parallel to your body.

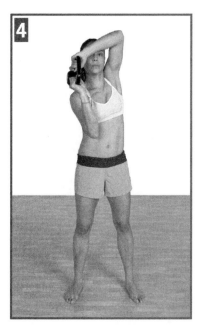

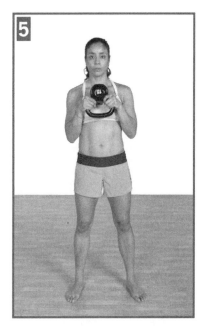

4 Continue rotating through the shoulders and pull the bell toward your right shoulder and your left forearm over your head.

5 As you bring the bell over your right shoulder and to the front and your left forearm clears your head, contract your abs and pull the bell down into starting position.

Derived from groundfighting-based martial arts, the Sit-Through is a bit more difficult than some of the other warm-ups but is great for warming up the core, upper body and hips. Plus it requires concentration and teaches you to move in a different way than most other bodyweight exercises.

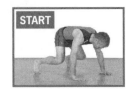
START

STARTING POSITION: Assume the quad position (hands on the floor a little wider than shoulder width and in the same plane as your shoulders; elbows bent slightly and angled out about 45 degrees from the rear; knees directly under your hips or slightly forward; feet same distance apart as your hands; back flat), keeping on the balls of your feet.

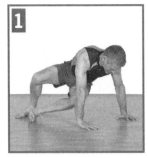

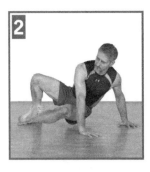

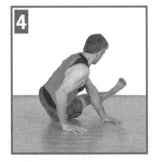

1–2 Rotate your hips to the right and at the same time pivot on your right foot so that your heel is down and your toes point directly to the right with your right knee up, shin vertical. Extend your left leg to the right, in front of your right leg but behind your arms. (You may lift your right hand off the floor, but keeping your hand on the floor works the core more.) Keep your left foot off the floor and your knee straight; your left leg should be at a 90-degree angle to your hands.

3 Pivot on your right foot and pull your left leg back under you to return to starting position. Adjust your hands and feet if necessary before doing a rep on the other side.

4 Repeat to the other side.

Cool-Downs

Cool-downs are an important part of your workout, and you should focus on them as much as every other aspect of your training. Properly cooling down helps you recover more quickly, improves your flexibility, prevents soreness and generally helps you re-energize yourself, particularly after a tough workout. There are hundreds of stretches and variations you can do, from the standard seated toe touch stretches for the hamstrings and lower back to advanced yoga poses, which can be as tough as the workout for some people.

We're going to focus on what I feel are the key stretches to compensate for the tension chains created by lifting kettlebells. Any exercise will tighten up your muscles—that's the "firm and tone" aspect of how most women train these days. But when you actually strength-train (which means lifting heavy, maxing out the weight you use in a few reps), stretching becomes especially important to help prevent the body from tightening up too much or in the wrong ways. Many of the stretches in this book will be familiar to you if you've done yoga or if you've read my previous book, *Spartan Warrior Workout* (Ulysses Press, 2010).

When you get this down, both shoulders should move at the same time but about half a movement apart. So while one shoulder is moving forward and down, the other is moving from the rear over the top and forward.

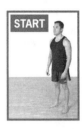

STARTING POSITION: Stand tall with your feet roughly shoulder-width apart and your arms relaxed by your sides, palms facing your thighs.

1 Roll your left shoulder up, backward, down and return it to its starting point. Try to do this slowly and smoothly.

2 Repeat with your right shoulder.

3 Now roll your left shoulder forward then down, pull it back to the rear, then up and over to return to the starting point.

4 Repeat with your right shoulder.

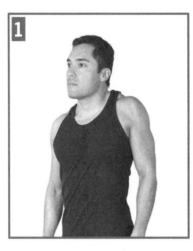

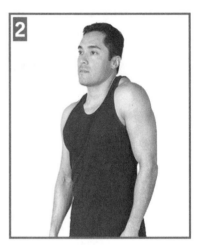

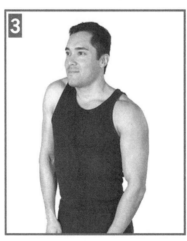

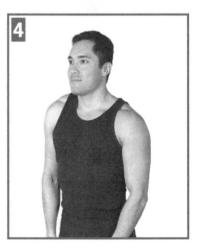

SHOULDER ROLL—DOUBLE

STARTING POSITION: Stand tall with your feet roughly shoulder-width apart and your arms relaxed by your sides, palms facing your thighs.

1 Roll both shoulders forward, then down, then pull them both back to the rear and up over the top to return to starting position.

2 Now lift both shoulders, pull them back and down, then roll them to the front to return to starting position.

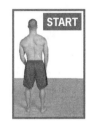

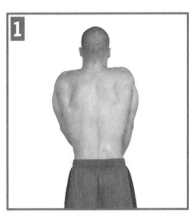

CHEST STRETCH

THE POSITION: Stand tall, reach both arms behind you and interlace your fingers. Straighten your elbows if you can, stick your chest out and pull your shoulders back. If you can straighten your elbows, try to lift your arms a little higher behind you.

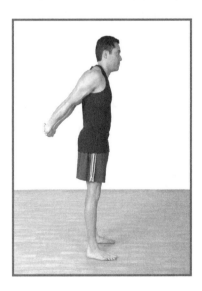

DOORWAY CHEST STRETCH

Using a doorway or having something to lean against and into will help open the chest and stretch the shoulders.

THE POSITION: Stand inside a doorway. Keeping your elbow straight, place your right arm on the outside of the door perpendicular to the floor. Keeping your arm in place, lean into the doorway. You can change the intensity and location of the stretch by lifting/lowering your arm higher/lower and also rotating it so that your palm is either against the wall or facing away from it.

Repeat on the other side.

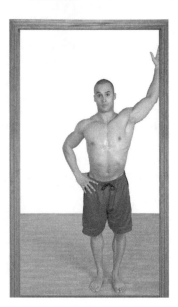

TRICEPS/SHOULDER STRETCH

THE POSITION: Stand tall. Take your right arm behind you and try to place the back of your hand on your left shoulder blade. Your palm will face away from your body. If you can't get your hand on your shoulder blade, you'll need to use a towel (see variation). Reach your left arm up and over your left shoulder, palm facing your back, and try to hook the fingers of both hands together.

Repeat on the other side.

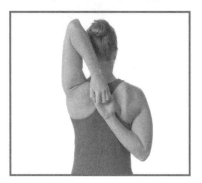

VARIATION: If you can't hook your fingers together, hold a towel in your high hand. Grab the towel in your low hand and walk the low hand up the towel as far as you can with minimal discomfort. Pull up with the high hand, opening the low hand's shoulder, and hold for 1 count. Pull down with the low hand to stretch the left triceps, holding for 1 count. Repeat this 5 times each way.

DOWNWARD DOG

This classic yoga pose opens the shoulders and chest and stretches the calves and hamstrings.

THE POSITION: Assume a high plank and then drive your hips up and back, pushing back hard with your arms so that your head is between your arms but not hanging down; maintain a straight spine. From here, drive your heels toward the floor but don't let them actually touch it; if they do, move your feet back until your heels no longer touch the floor. You should feel a stretch in your calves and, if tight, your hamstrings and glutes.

If you aren't feeling a stretch in the calves, adjust your foot position. This is an active pose so don't stay relaxed—push. Hold the pose for 5 seconds.

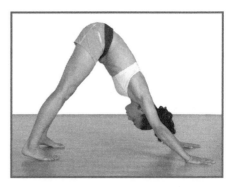

UPWARD DOG

Another classic yoga pose, this will help open the chest, lower back and hip flexors. If you're in Downward Dog, simply drop your hips to the floor, drive your shoulders down, lift your chest and bring your head up. Otherwise, follow these steps.

THE POSITION: Lie on your stomach with your hands roughly beside your ribs and your fingers pointing forward; keep your elbows by your sides. Extend your legs behind you with the tops of your feet on the floor. Push the ground away, straightening your arms completely, so that only your palms and tops of your feet are on the floor. Reach your chest forward and up, keeping your shoulders down and away from your ears. Tilt your head back slightly, making sure not to crunch the back of your neck. Squeeze your glutes and press your pelvis to the floor. Hold the pose for 5 seconds.

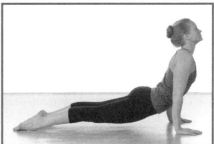

This yoga pose stretches your lats and lower back.

THE POSITION: Kneel with your feet together and knees slightly apart; the tops of your feet are on the floor. Sit your butt back on your heels and reach your arms as far forward as possible, palms facing down; keep your butt on your feet throughout the pose. Without moving your hands, lower your forearms to the floor. Hold for 5 seconds.

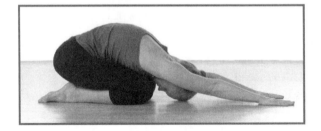

FIGURE 4

THE POSITION: Stand on your left leg with your knee straight. Bring your right foot up and place its outside edge above your left knee—the higher up the left thigh the better, as long as there is no discomfort, especially in the knee. Try to hold your right foot with your left hand, but maintain a tall spine—don't bend to reach your foot. Push your hips forward and pull your right knee back as far as you can without discomfort. Hold for 5 seconds, then repeat on the other side.

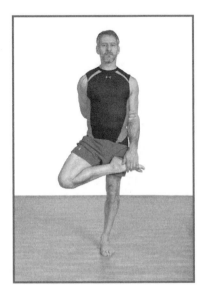

SQUATTING FIGURE 4

This stretch targets the side of both hips (gluteus medius and piriformis).

THE POSITION: Stand tall on your left leg. Bring your right foot up and place it on your left thigh just above your knee. Squat as deeply as you can; you can hold your arms in front of you for balance.

Repeat on the other side.

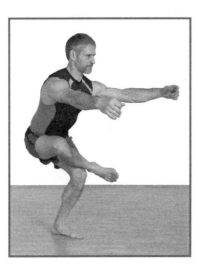

MODIFICATION: Lie on the floor on your back. Bend your right knee about 90 degrees and place your right foot just above your left knee. Keeping your right foot in place, pull your left knee toward your chest. Thread your right arm through the opening between your right and left legs and grab your left knee with your right hand; grab your left knee with your left hand as well. Use both hands to pull your knee to your chest, trying to keep the lower part of your left leg parallel to the floor.

SEATED HAMSTRING AND LOWER BACK STRETCH

This targets the hamstrings and lower back. Many people do this stretch improperly, usually by trying to get their head on their thighs or knees and thus rounding their back.

THE POSITION: Sit on the floor with your legs extended in front of you, knees straight. Your feet should be in line with your hips, not together or spread wide. Keeping your chest out, fold through your hips and reach out with your hands as far as you can. Try to grab your toes or ankles (see modification below if you have trouble with either) then pull with your arms. The goal is to get your chest to your feet. Don't bend through your back—focus on moving your chest toward your toes and keeping your shoulders pulled back. Don't look down at your legs—look out in front of you. Hold for 2 or 3 seconds, release and repeat 5 times. Try to go a little deeper into the stretch each time.

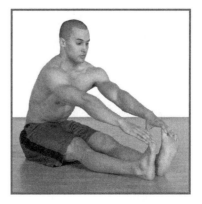

MODIFICATION: If you can't reach your ankles, place a towel around the bottoms of your feet and hold the ends. Now pull with your arms.

If you don't feel the stretch in your hip while keeping your butt cheeks flat on the floor, try the advanced variations.

THE POSITION: Sit on the floor with your legs extended in front of you, torso vertical. Your right hand is on the floor behind and slightly to the right of you; keep your elbow straight. Drive your right shoulder into the floor to keep your torso upright. Keeping both butt cheeks on the floor, place your right foot on the outside of your left thigh. Turn your torso to the right and wrap your left arm around your right knee. Continue to sit up tall. Hold for 5 seconds.

Repeat on the other side.

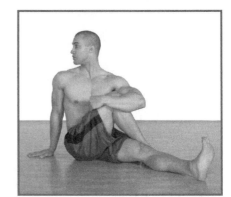

VARIATION 1: Instead of wrapping your arm around your knee, place the back of your arm on the outside of the opposite upright knee, elbow straight and palm facing away. Pull the arm into the side of the leg to work the hip more.

VARIATION 2: Instead of keeping one leg straight, bend the knee and bring the foot under you. Perform either the basic seated twist or Variation 1. Just make sure your butt is on the ground and you're sitting upright.

VARIATION 3: To add on to Variation 2, reach your front arm over your front leg and then reach back through under your knee. If you're extremely limber, you can reach behind you with your other hand and try to bring your hands together.

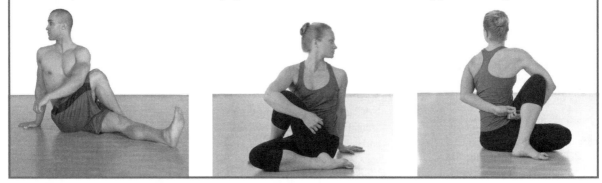

References

WEBSITES

Art of Strength (www.artofstrength.com): This site features kettlebell training information, equipment and Anthony DiLuglio's top-notch videos (some of the best follow-along workouts around).

Dragon Door (www.dragondoor.com): You'll find several of Pavel Tsatsouline's books here (*Enter the Kettlebell*, *The Russian Kettlebell Challenge*), as well as a forum, top-of-the-line kettlebells and other products.

International Kettlebell and Fitness Federation (www.ikff.net): This site has kettlebell training information and products, including several excellent kettlebell and bodyweight DVD sets by Steve Cotter.

Mahler's Aggressive Strength (www.mikemahler.com): This site provides kettlebell training DVDs as well as information on hormone optimization.

Max Condition (www.maxcondition.com): Jamie Hale's site offers great information on all aspects of training. You can also get his book *Knowledge and Nonsense: The Science of Nutrition and Exercise* here.

Perform Better (www.performbetter.com): This online store has kettlebells, bands, ropes and anything else you might need to strengthen your body.

RMAX International (www.rmaxinternational.com): This site promotes Scott Sonnon's joint mobility, Prasara Yoga, clubbells and bodyweight systems.

BOOKS

Jamie Hale, *Knowledge and Nonsense: The Science of Nutrition and Exercise*. Available at MaxCondition.com.

Dr. Mel Siff, *Facts and Fallacies of Fitness*. Available at EliteFTS.com.

Dr. Mel Siff, *Supertraining*. A must-read for the serious trainee or trainer. Available at EliteFTS.com.

Index

A

Advanced level, 16
    exercises, 86–109
    workouts, 24, 31–32, 34–35
Alternating cleans, 91–93
Armbar, 102

B

Beginner level, 16
    workouts, 24–28, 34–35
Bells, getting into position, 38–39, 50,
    73, 83–84
Biathlon, 10
Bodybuilding, 23
    history, 9
Bootstrapper, 117
Burpee Level 1, 116
Burpee Level 2, 116
Burpee Level 3, 117

C

Chalk, 89
Chest Stretch, 131
Cleans progressions, 49–58
Conditioning workouts, 26–27, 30, 31,
    32, 34–35
Conditioning, 18, 20
Cool-downs, 129–36

D

Dead Clean, 52–53
Dead Snatch, 86–87
Deadlift progressions, 64–69
Doorway Chest Stretch, 132
Double Dead Clean, 56
Double Hang Clean, 57
Double Pendulum Clean, 58
Double Swing, 48
Double Windmill, 106
Downward Dog, 133

E

Exercises, 38–109
    workout charts, 24–35

F

Figure 8, 79
Figure 8 with a Tap, 80–81
Figure 8s, 79–81
Figure Four, 134
Floor Press, 75–76
Forward Lunge, 122
Front Squat, 74

G

Getup Sit-Up, 101
Girevoy Sport (GS), 10, 83
Gloves, 84
Goblet Squat, 72–73
Golfers, 23

H

Half Getup, 96–97
Halo, 126–27
Hand care, 84
"Hand style," 83
Hand-to-Hand (H2H) Swing, 45
Hand-to-Hand (H2H) Swing with
    Release, 46
Handles, 13
Hang Clean, 54
Hang Snatch, 88
High Plank: Static Hold, 113
High Pull, 47

I

Intensity, 17, 19
Intermediate level, 16
    workouts, 24, 29–30, 34–35
Intervals and interval training, 17,
    19, 20

J

Jerks, 19, 107–108
Jogging, 9
Jumping Jacks, 119

K

KB sport, 10
Kettlebell training
    benefits, 11
    and existing routines, 23
    form and technique, 18, 22
    goals, 17
    history, 9
    intensity, 18, 21–22
    levels, 16
    preliminaries, 12–13
    programs, 16–35
    safety issues, 16
    workout charts, 24–35
Kettlebells
    handles, 13
    selection, 12
    styles and sizes, 12–13

L

Ladders, 20
Levels, 16
Lockout, 83
Low Plank: Static Hold, 113
Low Windmill, 104

M

Middle Plank: Static Hold, 113
Mountain Climber, 115

O

One-Arm Jerk, 108–109
One-Arm Vertical High Pull (1AVHP), 51
One-Hand Swing, 43–44
One-Leg Stiff-Leg Reach, 125
One-Leg Suitcase Deadlift, 66–67

One-Step Alternating Clean, 93
Overhead Press, 60–61
Overhead presses, 59–62
Overhead Windmill, 105

P

Partial Lower from High Plank, 114
Partial Raise from Low Plank, 114
Pendulum Clean, 55
Pendulum Snatch, 89–90
Planks, 113–14
Powerlifters, 23
Programs, 16–35
    designing, 17–29
    levels, 16
Push Press, 62–63
Push-Up, 112

R

Rack position, 50
Rate of Perceived Discomfort (RPD),
    21–22
Rate of Perceived Exertion (RPE), 21,
    22
Rate of Perceived Technique (RPT), 17,
    21, 22
Renegade Row, 82, 115
Reps, 17, 19–20
Rows, 77

S

Safety issues, 16
Seated Hamstring and Lower Back
    Stretch, 135
Seated Twist, 136
Sets, 17, 19–20
Shoulder Roll—Alternating, 130
Shoulder Roll—Double, 131
Side-to-Side Stepping Lunge, 121
Side-to-Side Stretch Lunge, 120
Sit-Through, 128
Sleeping Warrior, 134
Slingshots, 78
Snatches, 19, 83–90
Sonnon, Scott, 22
Spiderman Crawl, 118
Squat, 123
Squat progressions, 70–74
Squatting Figure Four, 135
Static Lunge, 123
Stiff-Legged One-Leg Deadlift, 68–69
Strength workouts, 28–29, 33
Stretching, 18, 129–36
Suitcase Deadlift, 65
Sumo Deadlift, 40–41
Sumo Squat, 71
Supersets, 20
Swing Snatch. *See Pendulum Snatch*
Swing progressions, 19, 38–48

T

Timed intervals, 17, 20
Training methods, history, 9
Tri-athletes, 23
Triceps/Shoulder Stretch, 132
Tri-sets, 20
Turkish Getup, 98–100
Turkish Getups (TGU), 94–102
    spotter directions, 95
Two-Hand Swing, 42
Two-Step Alternating Clean, 92

U

Upward Dog, 133

W

Warm-Ups, 18, 112–28
Weight lifting gloves, 84
Windmills, 103–106
Women, and kettlebell competitions,
    10
Workouts, 17–19
    charts, 24–35
    exercises, 24–35
    and existing routines, 23
    length, 22

Y

Yoga poses, 133, 134

Other Ulysses Press Books

Spartan Warrior Workout: Get Action-Movie Ripped in 30 Days

Dave Randolph, $14.95

In just one month, the high-intensity workouts in this book can give you the jaw-dropping physique of history's greatest soldiers. *Spartan Warrior Workout* takes you from merely being in shape to having the strength and endurance to withstand the ultimate test.

7 Weeks to 50 Push-Ups: Strengthen and Sculpt Your Arms, Shoulders, Back and Abs by Training to Do 50 Consecutive Pull-Ups

Brett Stewart, $14.95

Most people don't realize that the time-honored pull-up is an incredibly effective and efficient workout for the entire upper body. Use the specially designed program in this book and you will go from doing just one pull-up to performing 50 consecutive reps—in the process transforming and building your biceps, shoulders, back and abs.

7 Weeks to 100 Push-Ups: Strengthen and Sculpt Your Arms, Abs, Chest, Back and Glutes by Training to Do 100 Consecutive Push-Ups

Steve Speirs, $14.95

If you're ready to massively increase your strength, follow the book's 7-week program and you'll soon be able to complete 100 consecutive push-ups! You'll also transform your fitness, look great and feel even better as you sculpt every muscle from your neck down to your calves.

Black Belt Krav Maga: Elite Techniques of the World's Most Powerful Combat System

Darren Levine & Ryan Hoover, $15.95

As the official defensive tactics system of Israeli police, military and elite special operations units, Krav Maga has proven its effectiveness. For the first time, *Black Belt Krav Maga* teaches and illustrates the discipline's most lethal fighting and self-defense moves in book format.

Complete Krav Maga: The Ultimate Guide to Over 230 Self-Defense and Combative Techniques

Darren Levine & John Whitman, $21.95

Developed for the Israel military forces, Krav Maga is an easy-to-learn yet highly effective art of self-defense. Clearly written and extensively illustrated, *Complete Krav Maga* details every aspect of the system, including hand-to-hand combat moves and weapons defense techniques.

Corps Strength: A Marine Master Gunnery Sergeant's Program for Elite Fitness

MGySgt. Paul J. Roarke, $14.95

Renowned for its rigorous fitness training, the Marine Corps requires every member to be physically fit, regardless of age, grade or duty assignment. *Corps Strength* applies the same techniques used to develop and maintain each Marine's combat readiness to a day-to-day program for top-level fitness.

Dynamic Stretching: The Revolutionary New Warm-up Method to Improve Power, Performance and Range of Motion

Mark Kovacs, $14.95

Many top athletes and trainers have abandoned static stretching in favor of dynamic stretching. Now *Dynamic Stretching* teaches athletes and exercise enthusiasts everything they need to know about this breakthrough in sports performance.

Functional Training for Athletes at All Levels: Workouts for Agility, Speed and Power

James C. Radcliffe, $15.95

Teaches all athletes the functional training exercises that will produce the best results in their sport by mimicking the actual movements they utilize in that sport. With these unique programs, athletes can simultaneously improve posture, balance, stability and mobility.

Plyometrics for Athletes at All Levels: A Training Guide for Explosive Speed and Power

Neal Pire, $15.95

Provides the nonprofessional with an easy-to-understand explanation of why plyometrics works, the sports-training research behind it, and how to integrate plyometrics into an overall fitness program.

Total Heart Rate Training: Customize and Maximize Your Workout Using a Heart Rate Monitor

Joe Friel, $15.95

Shows anyone participating in aerobic sports, from novice to expert, how to increase the effectiveness of his or her workout by utilizing a heart rate monitor.

To order these books call 800-377-2542 or 510-601-8301, fax 510-601-8307, e-mail ulysses@ulyssespress.com, or write to Ulysses Press, P.O. Box 3440, Berkeley, CA 94703. All retail orders are shipped free of charge. California residents must include sales tax. Allow two to three weeks for delivery.

Acknowledgments

Many thanks to family and friends, who continually push me to learn and grow, encourage me to follow my dreams and give me the support to keep forging ahead. To Cheryl—if it weren't for you, I wouldn't be where I am today; thanks for your love and support. Special thanks to Pat and Holly Rigsby for their support and mentoring. To Pavel Tsatsouline, Steve Cotter, Scott Sonnon and the people in their respective organizations, who have all taught me a lot about kettlebells and training in general. To Lily, Claire and the rest of the staff at Ulysses Press, for the great work they did in editing and producing this book.

About the Author

DISCARD

Dave Randolph, author of *Spartan Warrior Workout*, has been involved in martial arts since 1989, earning the rank of Master, 6th-degree black belt, in 2005. Through his martial arts training and teaching, Dave became interested in teaching fitness to more than just martial artists. In 2002, he became certified as a kettlebell instructor under Pavel Tsatsouline, who brought kettlebells into the mainstream around 1998. In 2007, he began teaching fitness at the only full-time kettlebell-centric gym in Louisville, Kentucky. Since then, Dave's unique methods have helped thousands of people become healthier and fitter.

Dave has studied kettlebells under several highly regarded kettlebell instructors and is constantly seeking to learn from the best in all fields in order to improve himself and what he teaches. By integrating joint mobility, strength, agility, flexibility and coordination, Dave's constantly evolving IronBody Fitness shows people how to elevate their health, fitness levels and quality of life.

If you'd like Dave to teach kettlebells in your area, or if you're a fitness professional looking to become a top-notch certified kettlebell instructor, visit Dave's website, www.iron-body.com, or kbuniversity.com.